# Power Pressure Cooker XL Cookbook

*5 Ingredients or Less – Easy and Delicious Electric Pressure Cooker Recipes For The Whole Family*

# TABLE OF CONTENTS

**Introduction** ............................................................................................................ 6
**Chapter 1: what is a Power Pressure Cooker XL?** ........................................... 7
    How it works ......................................................................................................... 7
        The PPC-XL features............................................................................................ 7
**Chapter 2: why use the Power Pressure Cooker XL?** ..................................... 10
    Saves time............................................................................................................. 10
    Less dishes to wash .............................................................................................. 10
    Keeps nutrients in the food.................................................................................. 10
    Faster "slow" cooking .......................................................................................... 10
    Infuses food with more flavor.............................................................................. 10
    Less cumbersome cooking ................................................................................... 10
**Chapter 3: Pressure Cooking Tips** ..................................................................... 11
    Remove steam and pressure safely ..................................................................... 11
    Don't overfill the pot ........................................................................................... 11
    Remember to use liquid ....................................................................................... 11
    Use a steaming basket.......................................................................................... 11
    Do not add thickeners to the pressure cooker .................................................... 11
**Chapter 4: Power Pressure Cooker XL Recipes** .............................................. 12
    **Tips and notes about these recipes** ................................................................. 12
        A note on timing: ................................................................................................ 12
        Ingredients: .......................................................................................................... 12
        Measurements:..................................................................................................... 12
    **Breakfast** ........................................................................................................... 13
        Apple and cinnamon oatmeal............................................................................. 13
        Potato, bacon, and egg hash ............................................................................... 14
        Stewed fruits with vanilla and almond................................................................ 15
        Creamy spinach and mushrooms ....................................................................... 16
        Breakfast beans ................................................................................................... 17
        Haloumi and bacon with baby spinach .............................................................. 18
        Mini quiches ........................................................................................................ 19
        Healthy 4-ingredient pancakes ........................................................................... 20
        Hard boiled eggs ................................................................................................. 21
        French toast......................................................................................................... 22
        "Caramel" banana oatmeal ................................................................................. 23
        Apple breakfast crumble..................................................................................... 24
        Fried vegetables with runny-yolk eggs ............................................................... 25
        Smoked salmon and egg muffins ....................................................................... 26
        Raspberry and pear breakfast topping............................................................... 27
        Sweet corn fritters............................................................................................... 28
        Toasted muesli .................................................................................................... 29
    **Soups and Stews** .............................................................................................. 29

- Smooth butternut pumpkin soup .................................................................. 30
- Leek and potato soup ..................................................................................... 31
- Chicken and corn chowder ............................................................................. 32
- Warming lamb stew ........................................................................................ 33
- Beef and potato stew ...................................................................................... 34
- Spicy capsicum and cumin soup .................................................................... 35
- White bean soup ............................................................................................. 36
- Spiced lamb and chickpea stew ..................................................................... 37
- Creamy mushroom soup ................................................................................. 38
- Parsnip and cauliflower soup ......................................................................... 39
- Coconut carrot soup ....................................................................................... 40
- Easy noodle soup ............................................................................................ 41
- Pressure cooker sausage stew ....................................................................... 42
- Minced lamb and tomato "stili" (stew and chili) ............................................ 43
- Ham hock soup ................................................................................................ 44
- Pork and apple stew ....................................................................................... 45
- Beef and onion stew with wine ...................................................................... 46

## Vegan and Vegetarian ..................................................................................... 46
- Vegetarian chili (V, VG) .................................................................................. 47
- Vegetarian fried rice (V) ................................................................................. 48
- Ginger, garlic, and honey tofu (V) ................................................................. 49
- Sweet potato salad (V) ................................................................................... 50
- Couscous, carrot, and seed salad (V) ............................................................ 51
- Spinach risotto (V) .......................................................................................... 52
- Spiced lentil soup (V, VG) ............................................................................... 53
- Creamy vegetable curry (V, VG) .................................................................... 54
- Avocado and capsicum sushi (VG, V) ............................................................ 55
- Brown rice, cashew, and broccoli salad (VG, V) ............................................ 56
- Vegetarian burger patties (V, VG) ................................................................. 57
- Olive and tomato spaghetti (V, VG) ............................................................... 58
- Lemon, pea, and parmesan penne pasta (V) ................................................ 59
- Refried beans (V, VG) ..................................................................................... 60
- Crispy eggplant dippers (V) ........................................................................... 61
- Rice noodles with cucumber, carrot, and sesame seeds (VG, V) ................. 62
- Pumpkin, peanut, and coconut side dish (VG, V) ......................................... 63

## Meat ................................................................................................................... 63
- Roast chicken .................................................................................................. 64
- Roast beef ....................................................................................................... 65
- Pork belly ........................................................................................................ 66
- PPC-XL chili .................................................................................................... 67
- Honey-glazed chicken drumsticks ................................................................. 68
- Rare steak strips with buttered corn ............................................................. 69
- Spicy coriander chicken ................................................................................. 70
- Pork and chive meatballs ............................................................................... 71

- Slow cooked lamb leg ... 72
- Pork chops with lemon zest ... 73
- Crumbed chicken ... 74
- Beef stir fry with garlic and soy ... 75
- Creamy lemon chicken ... 76
- Sausage and potato bake ... 77
- Spicy pork rice bowl ... 78
- Beef and bean burger patties ... 79

**Seafood** ... 79
- Simple sautéed sesame salmon ... 80
- Crispy crumbed fish with lemon mayonnaise ... 81
- White fish poached in tomato and olive sauce ... 82
- Lemon prawn starter snacks ... 83
- Spicy prawn ramen ... 84
- Fish cakes with parsley ... 85
- Fish stew ... 86
- Fish with lemon and coconut rice ... 87
- Easy tuna and pea pasta ... 88
- Steamed scallops ... 89
- Crab macaroni ... 90
- Golden rice with mixed seafood ... 91
- Mussels with garlic and wine ... 92
- Zesty cabbage and fish salad ... 93
- Hot, fresh salmon broth with Asian greens ... 94
- Mini fish tacos with minted yogurt ... 95

**Dessert** ... 95
- Chocolate pots ... 96
- Caramelized bananas and ice cream ... 97
- Vanilla custard ... 98
- Stewed stone fruits with cinnamon and vanilla ... 99
- Rice pudding ... 100
- Simple cheesecake ... 101
- Citrus pie ... 102
- Salted caramel sauce ... 103
- Ginger pudding ... 104
- Pear crumble ... 105
- Baked apples ... 106
- Lemon curd (for drizzling and topping) ... 107
- Mini berry cheesecakes ... 108

**Conclusion** ... 109
**Resources:** ... 109

# Introduction

Hello food lovers! Welcome to the 'Power Pressure Cooker XL Cookbook – 5 ingredients or less'. As you can already tell… this book is all about a very special appliance… the *Power Pressure Cooker XL*, (or "PPC-XL" as it's sometimes called here).

The Power Pressure Cooker XL is an extremely versatile and easy-to-use pressure cooker, with a whole range of functions which we will cover later in the book.

First, we cover the basic ins and outs of the Power Pressure Cooker XL, including; how it works, the features and functions, and how to use each button. We then move on to some key benefits of using this handy little gem, and some secret tricks and tips for pressure-cooking.

Then comes the best part, the recipes! All of these recipes have been formulated especially for the Power Pressure Cooker XL. Each recipe contains no more than 5 key ingredients, (not including pantry staples such as salt and pepper!), and are incredibly simple, fast, and fun to create.

# Chapter 1: what is a Power Pressure Cooker XL?

This is the "educational" section of the book, where you will learn *all* about your Power Pressure Cooker Xl, so by the time you get to the recipes, you'll be a total expert!

The Power Pressure Cooker XL is a digital pressure cooker with multiple functions and a removable, washable inner pot.

## How it works

In simple words: The Power Pressure Cooker XL uses high pressure and heat to infuse moisture into your food, along with intense flavors and juicy succulence. All you need to do is secure the lid, press a button, and walk away. Sounds too easy? Well, luckily for us…it is.

### *The PPC-XL features*

Manual steam release: The steam valve can be manually switched to "open", which immediately releases the steam. Or, you can allow the steam to be released naturally.

Safety-locked lid: The lid has been carefully designed to close and lock securely. Once the lid has been secured onto the pot, it will stay put until removed again. No need to worry about the lid flying off!

Large lid handle: The large handle makes releasing and locking the lid very safe and easy.

Non-stick pot: The inner pot of the Power Pressure Cooker XL is non-stick and durable. Simply remove it when you want to wash it, then put it back once it's clean and dry.

Stainless steel construction: The Power Pressure Cooker XL is made from sturdy stainless steel, which will last for a very long time, and will remain clean and tidy.

Digital display screen: The digital display screen clearly displays the time, function, and temperature information for simple and easy use.

Preset function buttons: The preset function buttons make cooking various dishes extremely easy. Each button has a default time setting, which can be adjusted with the press of a button.

The buttons and how to use them:

### *Delay timer*
Use this button to program the pot to begin cooking at a time of your choice. For example: you may want the pot to start cooking your stew an hour before you return home from work...simply program the pot to begin cooking at 4pm.

### *Canning/preserving*
This button is used for canning and preserving foods. You can make jams, chutneys, pickles... anything. The PPC-XL uses high pressure when the canning/preserving button is being used.

### *Soup/Stew*
Cook soups and stews for 10, 30, or 60 minutes.

### *Slow cook*
Slow cook your meat dishes for 2, 6, or 12 hours.

### *Rice/risotto*
You can cook any kind of rice with this function. Depending on what kind of rice you are using, select the 6, 18, or 25-minute time setting.

### *Beans/lentils*
Cook bean and lentil-based dishes for 5, 15, or 30 minutes.

### *Fish/Vegetables/Steam*
This function cooks fish and vegetables by steaming, to ensure they don't overcook. Cook for 2, 4, or 10 minutes. Use the steaming basket to place the food in, and be sure to pour at least 1 cup of water into the pot first.

### *Chicken/Meat*
Cook meat and poultry for 15, 40, or 60 minutes. You can use this button to sauté as well. Simply press the button and leave the lid off to sauté, simmer, and brown foods.

***Time adjustment***
This button allows you to adjust the time settings for each function.

***Keep warm/cancel***
When the allocated time for each cooking session finishes, the pot will automatically switch to "keep warm". Press this button if you want to remove the lid and access the food immediately after cooking. Press this button if you have pressed the wrong function button and need to start again.

# Chapter 2: why use the Power Pressure Cooker XL?

### Saves time

The PPC-Xl allows you to cook delicious meals in a fraction of the time. You don't need to attend to the pot while it cooks, or go through multiple cooking stages to achieve a dish. Eat great food without wasting time.

### Less dishes to wash

Throw the ingredients into the pot…press a button…enjoy. This sounds easy, right? It is. And you only have one pot to clean, the PPC-XL inner pot. Forget about piles of dishes taking up your kitchen bench!

### Keeps nutrients in the food

By cooking your food in the PPC-XL, you are keeping crucial nutrients in the food. Boiling food in water, (and other cooking methods), can actually deplete the food of the key nutrients, so by the time you eat it…it's just not as good!

### Faster "slow" cooking

Slow-cooked meals are delicious, but they can take a very long time, (obviously!). With the PPC-XL, you can achieve the taste and texture of slow-cooked meals, in a fraction of the time. Not only does this save time, but it conserves energy too.

### Infuses food with more flavor

The PPC-XL infuses meat and fish with ultimate flavor by locking the flavor into the pot, and circulating it through the food while it cooks. Never suffer through bland food again!

### Less cumbersome cooking

With the PPC-XL, you don't need to stand over a hot stove. You can press a button, and simply walk away until the pot has finished working its magic. The ease of this style of cooking is a great reason to try new and exotic dishes you may otherwise have avoided due to the effort required.

# Chapter 3: Pressure Cooking Tips

## Remove steam and pressure safely

If you choose to manually release the steam once your meal has finished cooking, remember to use a tea towel or cloth to protect your hand. Do not place your hand or arm directly over the steam valve.

## Don't overfill the pot

Overfilling the pot can result in bland and mushy food. Sometimes, overfilling the pot can actually stop the pot from reaching maximum pressure, which can mean your food comes out unevenly cooked. Only fill the pot half way.

## Remember to use liquid

If you don't add any liquid to the pot, you can risk burning the food. What's more, the pot needs liquid in order to create steam, which creates the even and moist result. Aim for at least 1 cup of liquid per dish.

## Use a steaming basket

When steaming vegetables or fish, use a steaming basket. This keeps the food away from the liquid directly, but allows the steam to cook and infuse the food without draining the nutrients.

## Do not add thickeners to the pressure cooker

If you add thickeners such as corn-starch or roux (butter and flour mixture) to the pressure cooker, the amount of steam created can be compromised, so you might end up with a dry or gluggy dish. If you want to use thickeners, stir them through the dish after the pressure cooker has finished cooking.

# Chapter 4: Power Pressure Cooker XL Recipes

## Tips and notes about these recipes

### *A note on timing:*

I have provided an approximate cooking time for each recipe. This time does not include the time it takes for the pot to reach pressure or temperature. The time refers to the total preparation and cooking time, once the pot has reached the required pressure and temperature.

### *Ingredients:*

Most of these ingredients are very easy to find at your local supermarket, even if they sound exotic! I have not included oil, salt, or pepper into the ingredients list, as I assume that everyone has these staples in their cupboards. These recipes are very forgiving, and you are totally welcome to modify the quantities according to how many people you are serving. You can also swap certain ingredients for other ingredients according to what's available to you. For example; you don't have limes? No problem! Just use lemons. You don't have the specific spices I have listed in the ingredients list? No problem! Use any similar spices you have, according to your taste preferences.

### *Measurements:*

Most recipes in the first 5 recipe sections use pounds as the main measurement. However, the recipes in the dessert section primarily use grams, as I believe that grams are a more accurate measurement to use when dealing with baking or dessert ingredients, as they are usually required in smaller quantities.

# Breakfast

A great breakfast can brighten your day and give you the energy to live life to the fullest, all day long. Even if your mornings are a stressed-out, rushed, and frantic time, try to grab something to munch on as you run out the door. For this purpose, there are some really time-friendly recipes in this section. For more leisurely mornings, why not treat yourself to a decadent breakfast of French toast or fried haloumi? You'll find these tempting recipes here as well. Whether it's savory or sweet, the PPC-XL can take care of all your breakfast dishes!

### *Apple and cinnamon oatmeal*

*I love oatmeal in the morning, and it just so happens to be extremely nutritious and filling! Classic flavors of apple and cinnamon make this morning dish extra special.*

**Serves:** 2
**Time:** approximately 10 minutes

**Ingredients:**
- 1 ½ cup oats (quick or wholegrain, whatever you have on hand)
- 3 cups water
- 1 tsp cinnamon
- 1 apple (any kind but I use Granny Smith), grated
- Pinch of salt

**Method:**
1. Place the oats, water, salt, and cinnamon into the PPC-XL.
2. Press the RICE button and keep the time at the default 6 minutes.
3. Place the lid onto the pot and make sure the steam valve is closed.
4. Once the pot beeps, press CANCEL, which stops the warming function, carefully release the steam and remove the lid.
5. Stir the grated apple through the oatmeal.
6. Serve with a drizzle of honey or milk, whatever you like best!
7. ENJOY!

## *Potato, bacon, and egg hash*

*Carbs and bacon in the morning? Yes please! Sometimes it's necessary to have a breakfast like this to get through a particularly crazy day.*

**Serves:** 4
**Time:** approximately 20 minutes

**Ingredients:**
- 2 large potatoes (any kind works), chopped into cubes
- 5 rashers streaky bacon, roughly chopped into small pieces
- 4 eggs, lightly beaten
- 1 tbsp olive oil
- Salt and pepper to season

**Method:**
1. Place the potatoes into the PPC-XL and sprinkle them with salt.
2. Pour a cup of water over the potatoes.
3. Secure the lid onto the pot and make sure the steam valve is closed.
4. Press the SOUP/STEW button and keep the time at the default 10 minutes.
5. Once the pot beeps, carefully release the steam and remove the lid.
6. Remove the potatoes and keep to one side.
7. Remove any excess water from the pot.
8. Drizzle the olive oil into the pot and press the MEAT/CHICKEN button.
9. Once the oil is hot, add the bacon to the pot and sauté until crispy.
10. Add the potatoes to the pot and stir until coated in oil and bacon, sauté for 5 minutes until browned and crispy.
11. Move the bacon/potato mixture to one side of the pot and add the eggs.
12. Quickly scramble the eggs with a spatula until cooked to your liking (I like mine quite soft and "runny").
13. Remove all ingredients from the pot and serve on 4 plates.
14. ENJOY!

## *Stewed fruits with vanilla and almond*

*Stewed fruits are a wonderful addition to yoghurt, oatmeal, cereal...or even on their own! I love to have a bowl of this vanilla mixture in my fridge for mornings when I need something a little sweeter. If you don't have any of the fruits in this recipe, use any seasonal fruits you can find! Apples, berries, cherries, pears...they all work just fine. You can also use any other nuts you have as well, such as pecans would be lovely!*

**Serves:** makes 1 large bowl, about 6 servings
**Time:** approximately 15 minutes

**Ingredients:**
- 3 lb peaches and nectarines, cut into chunks
- 1 tbsp sugar
- 1 tbsp vanilla extract (or essence)
- ¼ cup sliced almonds
- 1 ½ cups water

**Method:**
1. Place the fruit, sugar, vanilla, and water into the pot and press the SOUP/STEW button, keep the time at the default 10 minutes.
2. Place the lid onto the pot and make sure the steam valve is closed.
3. Once the pot beeps, carefully release the pressure and remove the lid.
4. Stir the fruit mixture and add the almonds.
5. Serve over yoghurt, oatmeal, or on its own.
6. ENJOY!

## *Creamy spinach and mushrooms*

*This delicious, creamy dish is perfect for vegetarians, and pairs really well with toasted bread and of course...a strong coffee!*

**Serves:** 4
**Time:** approximately 10 minutes

**Ingredients:**
- 4 large handfuls of spinach, (I use baby spinach, but any kind works)
- 2 cups chopped mushrooms, (a mixture of brown and white is fine)
- 1 tbsp olive oil
- ½ cup heavy cream
- Salt and pepper

**Method:**
1. If you are using normal spinach (not baby), chop it into small pieces.
2. Pour the olive oil into the pot and press the CHICKEN/MEAT button.
3. Once the oil is hot, add the mushrooms and spinach and stir until coated in oil.
4. Sauté the vegetables until the spinach is welted and the mushrooms are browned.
5. Add the cream, stir through, and cook until thickened.
6. Stir through salt and pepper to your taste.
7. Serve alone or with toast.
8. ENJOY!

## *Breakfast beans*

*Beans are SO nutritious, filling, healthy, and affordable. I always have many cans of black beans and kidney beans in the cupboard, ready to be used in all kinds of ways. Breakfast beans are awesome as they pack your day full of energy.*

**Serves:** 4
**Time:** approximately 20 minutes

**Ingredients:**
- 2 cans beans – black, kidney, or both (approx. 900gm in total)
- 1 can chopped tomatoes
- 1 onion, finely chopped
- 1 tbsp olive oil
- 1 tsp chili powder

**Method:**
1. Place olive oil, onion, chili powder, tomatoes, and beans into the PPC-XL.
2. Press the BEANS/LENTILS button and adjust the time to 15 minutes.
3. Secure the lid onto the pot and make sure the steam valve is closed.
4. Once the pot beeps, carefully release the steam and remove the lid.
5. Stir the beans and serve with toast, eggs, or anything you wish! It's great on its own.
6. ENJOY!

## *Haloumi and bacon with baby spinach*

*Don't be afraid if you've never tried haloumi! You can get it in ALL supermarkets these days, in the cheese section. It's salty, creamy, and amazingly delicious.*

**Serves:** 2
**Time:** approximately 12 minutes

**Ingredients:**
½ block haloumi cheese, (about 150gm), cut into slices
4 rashers streaky bacon
2 large handfuls baby spinach
1 tbsp olive oil

**Method:**
1. Add the olive oil to the PPC-XL.
2. Press the CHICKEN/MEAT button.
3. Once the oil is hot, add the haloumi slices to the pot and fry on both sides until golden.
4. Remove the haloumi from the pot and place to one side on a plate.
5. Add the bacon to the pot and cook until crispy.
6. Remove the bacon from the pot and place to one side with the haloumi.
7. Add the spinach to the pot and stir until coated in the oil and bacon juices, sauté until wilted and soft.
8. Remove the spinach from the pot divide it into 2 and serve on a plate with haloumi and bacon.
9. ENJOY!

## *Mini quiches*

*These are part muffin, part quiche...ALL amazing. The steaming basket which comes with your Power Pressure Cooker XL comes in handy with this recipe. I like to have these on hand for weeks when I just know I won't have the time to cook a decent breakfast in the morning, as I can simply "grab one and go".*

**Serves:** makes 8 mini quiches
**Time:** approximately 10 minutes

### Ingredients:
- 5 eggs
- 3 tbsp milk
- 1 green onion, finely chopped
- 150g feta cheese, chopped into small chunks
- Fresh parsley, chopped (or any other fresh herb you have lying around!)

### Method:
1. Crack the eggs into a bowl; add the milk, chopped green onion, feta, and parsley.
2. With a fork, beat the mixture together until the eggs are beaten and smooth.
3. Pour about a cup of water into the bottom of the PPC-XL.
4. Place the steaming basket into the PPC-XL.
5. Place 8 cupcake cases into the steaming basket.
6. Pour the quiche mixture into the 8 cupcake cases.
7. Secure the lid onto the pot and make sure the steam valve is closed.
8. Press the FISH/VEG/STEAM button and adjust the time to 4 minutes.
9. Once the pot beeps, carefully release the steam and remove the lid, take out the quiches and leave to cool slightly before eating.
10. ENJOY!

## *Healthy 4-ingredient pancakes*

*Yes, you read that right...pancakes can be healthy! In fact, "healthy pancakes" are very popular these days, especially with fitness fanatics and gym bunnies. If you are craving something tasty and a little "treat-like", but don't want to compromise your healthy eating routine, then these are ideal for you.*

**Serves:** makes about 9 pancakes (about 3 servings)
**Time:** approximately 12 minutes

**Ingredients:**
- 1 large banana, mashed
- 2 eggs, lightly beaten
- ½ cup oats
- 1 tsp cinnamon
- Coconut oil for frying (or any other mild-flavored oil you have)

**Method:**
1. In a bowl, mix together the banana, egg, oats, and cinnamon until smooth and combined.
2. Drizzle some oil into the PPC-XL and press the CHICKEN/MEAT button.
3. Once the oil is hot, drop about 2tbsp mixture into the pot to create a pancake, make sure you don't overcrowd the pot, so do about 2 or 3 pancakes at the time.
4. Once you see bubbles appear on the top of the pancake, carefully flip it over and cook the other side until both sides are golden.
5. Serve with yoghurt, fruit, or anything your heart desires!
6. ENJOY!

## *Hard boiled eggs*

*As boring as this recipe might seem, hard boiled eggs can actually be a total life saver when life gets completely crazy. I often prepare a batch of hard boiled eggs on a Sunday night to keep in the fridge for the week. I grab one when I need a super-quick breakfast or a healthy snack.*

**Serves:** makes 10 hard-boiled eggs (but you can adjust this and make as many as you like)
**Time:** approximately 8 minutes

**Ingredients:**
- 10 eggs
- 2 cups water

**Method:**
1. Pour the water into the bottom of the pot.
2. Place the eggs into the steaming basket.
3. Place the basket into the pot.
4. Press the RICE/RISOTTO button and keep the time at the default 6 minutes.
5. Secure the lid onto the pot and make sure the steam vent is closed.
6. Once the pot beeps, carefully release the steam and remove the lid.
7. Leave the eggs to cool, and store in the fridge.
8. ENJOY!

## *French toast*

*Okay, seriously, who doesn't love French toast?! The Power Pressure Cooker XL makes the process so easy and quick, you can enjoy this tasty breakfast whenever you like! Old bread works just as well as fresh bread, so it's a great way of using up bread that would otherwise go to waste.*

**Serves:** 2
**Time:** approximately 10 minutes

**Ingredients:**
- 4 thick slices white bread
- 2 eggs, lightly beaten
- 2 tbsp milk
- 2 tbsp sugar
- 1 tsp cinnamon

**Method:**
1. In a bowl, mix together the beaten eggs and milk.
2. Sprinkle the sugar and cinnamon onto a plate and combine.
3. Dip the sliced bread into the milk/egg mixture so that both sides are coated.
4. Dip the coated bread into the sugar mixture so that each piece is lightly coated on both sides.
5. Add a drizzle of mild oil into the PPC-XL (coconut oil works well).
6. Press the CHICKEN/MEAT button.
7. Once the oil is hot, add 2 slices of coated bread at a time and cook on both sides until golden and crispy on the outside.
8. Serve the French toast however you like! Berries are a great topping.
9. ENJOY!

## *"Caramel" banana oatmeal*

*I just had to add another oatmeal recipe, as I just love oatmeal so much. This "caramel" oatmeal is not as unhealthy as it sounds, but it's definitely a luxurious breakfast treat.*

**Serves:** 2
**Time:** approximately 8 minutes

**Ingredients:**
- 1 ½ cup oats (quick or wholegrain)
- 1 cup full-fat milk
- 1 cup water
- 1 large banana, chopped into slices
- 1 tbsp brown sugar

**Method:**
1. Place the oats, milk, water, and brown sugar into the PPC-XL.
2. Secure the lid onto the pot and make sure the steam valve is closed.
3. Press the RICE button and keep the time at the default 6 minutes.
4. Once the pot beeps, carefully release the steam and remove the lid.
5. Stir the banana through the oatmeal so it warms through, and slightly "melts" into the oatmeal.
6. Serve with milk and an extra sprinkle of brown sugar.
7. ENJOY!

## *Apple breakfast crumble*

*Crumble for BREAKFAST? Yup, you bet. This crumble is less sugary and buttery than the usual dessert crumble, but it's just as good. Apples are one of the best creations under the sun, in my opinion, and once you add a topping of crunchy, nutty crumble...it's just heavenly.*

**Serves:** 4 or 5
**Time:** approximately 20 minutes

**Ingredients:**
- 4 granny smith apples, peeled and sliced
- 1 cup oats
- ½ cup shredded coconut
- ¼ cup chopped almonds
- 2tbsp butter, melted

**Method:**
1. Place the sliced apples into the bottom of the PPC-XL and add a sprinkling of water, (about 3 tablespoons).
2. In a bowl, mix together the oats, coconut, almonds, and melted butter until a crumble forms.
3. Sprinkle the crumble over the apples.
4. Secure the lid onto the pot and make sure the steam valve is closed.
5. Press the CHICKEN/MEAT button and keep the time to the default 15 minutes.
6. Once the pot beeps, carefully release the steam and remove the lid.
7. Serve the crumble in bowls with yoghurt, or any other breakfast accompaniments you like.
8. ENJOY!

## *Fried vegetables with runny-yolk eggs*

*Starting your day with vegetables is a fantastic way of ensuring you are getting enough nutrients into your diet. Adding an egg on top boosts your protein intake, and the runny yolk creates a saucy sensation.*

**Serves:** 4
**Time:** approximately 8 minutes

**Ingredients:**
- 1 cup chopped mushrooms
- 1 large zucchini, cut into small chunks
- 1 red capsicum, seeds removed and cut into small pieces
- 1tbsp olive oil
- 4 eggs, (1 egg per serving)

**Method:**
1. Pour the olive oil into the PPC-XL.
2. Press the CHICKEN/MEAT button.
3. Once the oil is hot, add the vegetables and sprinkle with salt and pepper if you wish.
4. Sauté the vegetables until soft and starting to brown.
5. Remove the vegetables from the pot.
6. Add the eggs one at a time to the pot and fry just enough to cook the whites, but keep the yolks runny and dark yellow.
7. Remove the eggs from the pot once they are cooked and place on top of the vegetables.
8. Serve while hot.
9. ENJOY!

## *Smoked salmon and egg muffins*

*Smoked salmon might seem indulgent, but it's available in every supermarket, and it's packed with Omega-3 fatty acids. These salmon and egg muffins are amazing for an easy breakfast or morning snack.*

**Serves:** makes 8 muffins
**Time:** approximately 10 minutes

**Ingredients:**
- 4 eggs, lightly beaten
- 2 tbsp full-fat milk or cream (whatever you've got)
- 75g smoked salmon, cut into small pieces
- Fresh chives, finely chopped
- Salt and pepper to taste

**Method:**
1. In a bowl, mix together the eggs, salmon, milk/cream, chives, salt, and pepper.
2. Pour 2 cups of water into the bottom of the PPC-XL.
3. Place the steaming basket into the pot.
4. Place 8 cupcake cases into the basket.
5. Fill each cupcake case with egg mixture.
6. Press the FISH/VEG/STEAM button and keep the time at the default 2 minutes.
7. Secure the lid onto the pot and make sure the steam valve is closed.
8. Once the pot beeps, carefully release the steam and remove the lid.
9. Leave the muffins to cool.
10. ENJOY!

## *Raspberry and pear breakfast topping*

*Raspberry and pear… what a phenomenal combination. When these gorgeous fruits are cooked in the Power Pressure Cooker XL, they become stew-like and perfect for dolloping on top of yoghurt, cereal, or oatmeal. You can even serve it on top of ice cream for dessert…*

**Serves:** makes one large bowl of topping, about 8 servings
**Time:** 15 minutes

**Ingredients:**
- 2 cups frozen raspberries
- 4 large pears, peeled, cored, and cut into chunks
- 1 tbsp sugar (or honey if you don't want to add refined sugar)
- 1 tbsp vanilla extract or essence
- ¾ cup water

**Method:**
1. Place the raspberries, pears, sugar/honey, vanilla, and water into the PPC-XL.
2. Press the SOUP/STEW button and keep the time at the default 10 minutes.
3. Secure the lid onto the pot and make sure the steam valve is closed.
4. Once the pot beeps, carefully release the steam and remove the lid.
5. Stir the fruit mixture and transfer it into a clean bowl,
6. Leave to cool before storing in the fridge, covered.
7. ENJOY!

## *Sweet corn fritters*

*I LOVE fritters, all kinds...but my favorite just has to be sweet corn. You can make these fritters the night before, store them in the fridge, then heat them under the grill in the oven when you need them. I like to serve mine with plain Greek yoghurt, and either bacon or salmon. You can serve yours however you wish!*

**Serves:** makes 12 fritters (3 or 4 servings)
**Time:** approximately 12 minutes

**Ingredients:**
- 3 cups corn kernels, (frozen or canned)
- 2 eggs, lightly beaten
- 3 tbsp self-raising
- 1 tbsp chopped fresh chives
- Salt and pepper

**Method:**
1. Combine corn, eggs, flour, chives, salt and pepper in a bowl.
2. Mix until the flour has been incorporated into the mixture and there are no lumps to be seen.
3. Press the CHICKEN/MEAT button on the PPC-XL.
4. Drizzle some oil into the pot, (any oil you have).
5. Once the oil is hot, place dollops of fritter batter into the pan (about 2tbsp each fritter).
6. Cook each side for about 2 mins or until each side is golden and crispy
7. Continue to cook fritters in batches of 4 or 5, until all mixture has been used up.
8. Serve with any sides or toppings you desire.
9. ENJOY!

## *Toasted muesli*

*To me, muesli is one of the most classic breakfast dishes. Eating a bowl of muesli with cold milk and some fresh fruit feels so wholesome and easy. It reminds me of when I used to eat cereal on Saturday mornings while watching cartoons on the TV! This recipe is healthy, easy, and lasts for weeks if you store in an airtight container.*

**Serves:** makes 1 large container of muesli
**Time:** 10 minutes

**Ingredients:**
- 4 cups oats, (wholegrain is best, but any you have is fine)
- ¼ cup desiccated coconut
- ½ cup dried apricots, chopped into small pieces
- ¼ cup seeds of your choice, (use a mixture of chia, pumpkin, sesame if you wish! But any will do)
- ¼ cup coconut oil, melted, (or any mild-taste oil you have such as sunflower or rice bran)

**Method:**
1. In a large bowl, place all ingredients and combine until incorporated and all dry ingredients covered with a light layer of oil.
2. Press the CHICKEN/MEAT button on your PPC-XL.
3. Once the pot is hot, add the muesli mixture and stir while it cooks and browns.
4. Remove the muesli once it is toasted, golden, and crunchy.
5. Place onto a baking sheet and leave to cool and become crunchy.
6. Transfer to an airtight container and store somewhere cool and dry.
7. Serve with milk, yoghurt, fruit… whatever you wish!
8. ENJOY!

# Soups and Stews

Soups and stews are the quintessential dish for Winter and Autumn. They are the best way to use up leftover or excess vegetables, as you can simply throw them in the PPC-X with some stock, press a button…and voila! Dinner. I have included a range of different soup and stew recipes in this section, including meaty stews and veggie-filled soups. Of course, I always serve my soup with crusty bread and butter! But that's up to you.

## *Smooth butternut pumpkin soup*

*What better recipe to start this section with than a classic, creamy, butternut pumpkin soup? I always find that butternut makes for a far better soup than regular crown pumpkin. Serve with buttery, crusty bread.*

**Serves:** about 6 medium servings
**Time:** 20 minutes

**Ingredients:**
- 1 large butternut pumpkin, peeled, deseeded, and chopped into cubes
- 1 onion, finely chopped
- 1 tbsp olive oil
- 1.5 liters chicken or vegetable stock
- 1 cup heavy cream

**Method:**
1. Place the olive oil into the PPC-XL.
2. Press the SOUP/STEW button and keep the lid off.
3. Once the oil is hot, add the onion and sauté until soft.
4. Add the butternut pumpkin and stock.
5. Add a pinch of salt and pepper.
6. Secure the lid onto the pot and make sure the steam valve is closed.
7. Press the keep the timer at the default 10 minutes.
8. Once the pot beeps, carefully release the steam and remove the lid.
9. With a hand-held stick blender, blend the soup until very smooth.
10. Stir the cream through the soup.
11. Serve white hot.
12. Enjoy!

## *Leek and potato soup*

*Leek and potato soup is the king of comforting soups. The onion-y goodness of the leeks gives the thick, creamy potatoes a gentle kick. You can make this healthier by swapping the cream for milk...but go on, use the cream!*

**Serves:** about 6 medium servings
**Time:** approximately 20 minutes

**Ingredients:**
- 4 lb potatoes, peeled and chopped into chunks
- 3 leeks, washed and roughly chopped
- 1 tbsp olive oil
- 1 1/2 liters chicken or vegetable stock
- 1 cup heavy cream

**Method:**
1. Press the SOUP/STEW button on your PPC-XL
2. Pour the oil into the pot
3. Once the oil is hot, add the leeks and sauté for a minute or two until slightly soft
4. Add the potatoes and stock.
5. Secure the lid onto the pot and make sure the steam valve is closed.
6. Keep the time at the default 10 minutes.
7. Once the pot beeps, carefully release the steam and remove the lid.
8. With a hand-held stick blender, blend until smooth.
9. Stir through the cream.
10. ENJOY!

## *Chicken and corn chowder*

*Chicken and corn, what a combination. This recipe uses left over chicken, which makes it so much easier! Of course, you can cook your chicken especially for this recipe, but I like to make this whenever I have left over roast chicken or some extra chicken breast or thigh.*

**Serves:** about 6 medium servings
**Time:** approximately 40 minutes

**Ingredients:**
- 2 cups shredded cooked chicken
- 2 cups corn kernels, (fresh, frozen, or canned)
- 1 onion, finely chopped
- 1 liter chicken stock
- 1 cup heavy cream

**Method:**
1. Place chicken, corn, onion, and stock into your PPC-XL.
2. Season with salt and pepper if you wish.
3. Press the SOUP/STEW button and adjust the time to 30 minutes.
4. Once the pot beeps, carefully release the steam and remove the lid.
5. Stir through the cream.
6. Serve while hot.
7. ENJOY!

## *Warming lamb stew*

*Lamb is such a great stewing meat. This classic, easy stew is simple yet utterly satisfying. Choose a cheap cut of lamb from your butcher such as shoulder, as it's ideal for slow cooking.*

**Serves:** about 5 large servings
**Time:** approximately 70 minutes

**Ingredients:**
- 4 lb lamb, cut into cubes and tossed in some flour (about ¼ cup)
- 1 large onion, finely chopped
- 4 carrots, chopped into chunks
- 3 tins chopped tomatoes
- 1 lamb stock cube, water

**Method:**
1. Press the SOUP/STEW button on your PPC-XL and do not put the lid on.
2. Once the pot is hot, drizzle some oil into the pot and add the floured lamb cubes, cook for a couple of minutes to brown the outside of the lamb.
3. Add the onion, tomatoes, carrots, stock cube, and about 1 cup of water.
4. Secure the lid onto the pot and make sure the steam valve is closed.
5. Adjust the time to 60 minutes.
6. Once the pot beeps, carefully release the steam and remove the lid.
7. Give the stew a stir, and serve while hot.
8. ENJOY!

## *Beef and potato stew*

*Beef and potato stew, it doesn't get much simpler than that! This is such an affordable stew to make, and it feeds up to 6 people on a budget, as you can get cheap cuts of stewing beef from the butcher. Serve with crusty bread and a side of buttered green beans...I'm hungry just writing this!*

**Serves:** about 6 medium servings
**Time**: approximately 70 minutes

**Ingredients:**
- 4 lb stewing beef, cut into cubes and tossed in some flour (about ¼ cup)
- 2 lb potatoes, skin on, cut into large chunks
- 2 onions, roughly chopped
- 2 liters beef stock (or 2 stock cubes and 2 liters of water)
- 1 tin chopped tomatoes

**Method:**
1. Press the SOUP/STEW button on your PPC-XL.
2. Drizzle some oil into the pot.
3. Add the floured beef to the pot and cook for about 2 minutes to brown the meat.
4. Add the potatoes, onions, stock, and tomatoes to the pot.
5. Season with salt and pepper.
6. Adjust the time to 60 minutes.
7. Once the pot beeps, carefully release the steam and remove the lid.
8. Serve while hot.
9. ENJOY!

## *Spicy capsicum and cumin soup*

Capsicums (sweet peppers) make for such a divine soup. If you like, you can throw them under the grill in the oven and cook them a bit before cooking in the PPC-XL, this gives them a roasted and slightly smoky flavor. However, for this recipe, we simply chuck them in the pot raw! So easy, so yummy.

**Serves:** about 6 medium servings
**Time:** approximately 20 minutes

**Ingredients:**
- 6-8 peppers (6 if large, 8 if small), seeded and roughly chopped
- 3 carrots, roughly chopped
- 1 onion, roughly chopped
- 1 heaped tsp ground cumin
- 1 ½ liters vegetable or chicken stock

**Method:**
1. Press the SOUP/STEW button on your PPC-XL and keep the time to the time to 10 minutes.
2. Drizzle some oil into the pot.
3. Once the oil is hot, add the onions, peppers, carrot, and cumin.
4. Sauté for a few minutes to combine the flavors and soften the onion.
5. Add the stock to the pot and secure the lid, make sure the steam valve is closed.
6. Once the pot beeps, carefully release the steam and remove the lid.
7. With a hand-held stick blender, blend until smooth.
8. If you like a creamier soup, you can add some cream or sour cream, but I like to keep this one a bit sharper!
9. ENJOY!

## *White bean soup*

*I am such a huge fan of beans! They are full of nutritional value, are incredibly affordable, and can be used in a multitude of ways. This recipe stars the under-looked white bean, (otherwise known as cannellini beans).*

**Serves:** about 6 medium servings
**Time:** approximately 20 minutes

**Ingredients:**
- 3 tins white beans, (about 2 ½ lb)
- 4 rashers streaky bacon, chopped into pieces
- 4 garlic cubes, finely chopped
- 1 liter vegetable or chicken stock
- ¾ cup full fat milk

**Method:**
1. Press the SOUP/STEW button on your PPC-XL.
2. Add the bacon to the pot and heat until the fat melts and the bacon is slightly crispy.
3. Add the garlic to the pot and heat until just beginning to soften.
4. Add the beans and stock to the pot.
5. Secure the lid onto the pot and make sure the steam valve is closed.
6. Keep the time to the default 10 minutes on the SOUP/STEW function.
7. Once the pot beeps, carefully release the steam and remove the lid.
8. With a potato masher, mash the soup so that it's creamy yet chunky.
9. Stir through the milk.
10. ENJOY!

## *Spiced lamb and chickpea stew*

*Yes, another lamb recipe! This one has the glorious addition of chickpeas to bulk it out and give it that nutty hum. Use tinned chickpeas instead of dried, it's far easier. The warm spices add a beautiful layer to this dish, which makes it a great choice for Winter or Autumn dinners. Use any savory spices you have, just make up a 2-teaspoon mixture of whatever is lurking in your cupboard.*

**Serves:** 4-6
**Time:** approximately 70 minutes

**Ingredients:**
- 4lb stewing lamb, diced and tossed in ¼ cup flour
- 1 onion, finely chopped
- 1 tin chickpeas
- 2tsp mixed spices: dried coriander, cumin, chili powder, garam masala, turmeric etc....
- 1 ½ liters beef stock, or 1 beef stock cube and 1 ½ liters water

**Method:**
1. Press the SOUP/STEW button and drizzle some oil into the pot.
2. Once the oil is hot, add the onion and spices, and sauté until soft.
3. Add the floured lamb and sauté for a few minutes until browned.
4. Add the chickpeas, stock, and water if using.
5. Secure the lid onto the pot and make sure the steam valve is closed.
6. Adjust the time for 60 minutes.
7. Once the pot beeps, carefully release the steam and remove the lid.
8. Give the stew a stir and serve while hot.
9. ENJOY!

## *Creamy mushroom soup*

*If you don't like mushrooms, then skip this recipe! If you love them? Then this soup might just be your new favorite. I like to use flat brown mushrooms, but a mixture of any mushrooms works just as well. This soup just screams for hot, buttered toast on the side, (you can tell by now that I love toast, can't you?).*

**Serves:** 6
**Time:** approximately 20 minutes

**Ingredients:**
- 2 lb mushrooms, roughly chopped
- 1 onion, roughly chopped
- 1 tbsp butter
- 1 ½ liters chicken stock
- ½ cup heavy cream

**Method:**
1. Press the SOUP/STEW button on your PPC-XL.
2. Add the butter to the pot, and once it has melted, add the onion and sauté until soft.
3. Add the mushrooms and sauté for 1 minute.
4. Add the stock and a pinch of salt and pepper.
5. Secure the lid onto the pot and keep the time at the default 10 minutes.
6. Once the pot beeps, carefully release the steam and remove the lid.
7. With a hand-held stick blender, blend until smooth.
8. Stir the cream through the soup.
9. Serve hot.
10. ENJOY!

## *Parsnip and cauliflower soup*

*I first tried a variation of this soup at my friend's house one night, her mother had made it and it was amazing. This version is just as good, and it's so easy and affordable to create.*

**Serves:** 6
**Time:** approximately 20 minutes

**Ingredients:**
- 1 cauliflower head, stalk and core removed, cut into florets
- 4 parsnips, peeled and cut into chunks
- 1 onion, roughly chopped
- 1 ½ liter chicken stock
- ½ cup heavy cream

**Method:**
1. Press the SOUP/STEW button on your PPC-XL and drizzle some oil into the pot.
2. Add the onion to the pot and sauté until soft.
3. Add the parsnip, cauliflower, stock, and a pinch of salt and pepper.
4. Secure the lid onto the pot and make sure the steam valve is closed.
5. Keep the time to the default 10 minutes.
6. Once the pot beeps, carefully release the steam and remove the lid.
7. With a hand-held stick blender, blend until very smooth.
8. Stir the cream through the soup and serve hot.
9. ENJOY!

## *Coconut carrot soup*

*Carrots are one of the most versatile vegetables, and they make a truly delicious soup. The coconut cream gives a slightly Thai flavor to this bright orange concoction. Serve with a sprinkling of fresh coriander if you like!*

**Serves:** 6
**Time:** approximately 40 minutes

**Ingredients:**
- 3 lb carrots, peeled and chopped into chunks
- 1 onion, roughly chopped
- 1 large potato, peeled and chopped
- 1 liter chicken stock
- 1 can coconut cream

**Method:**
1. Press the SOUP/STEW button on your PPC-XL and add a drizzle of oil to the pot.
2. Add the onion and sauté until soft.
3. Add the potato, carrot, stock, and a pinch of salt and pepper.
4. Secure the lid onto the pot and make sure the steam valve is closed.
5. Adjust the time to 30 minutes.
6. Once the pot beeps, carefully release the steam and remove the lid.
7. With a hand-held blender, blend until smooth.
8. Add the coconut cream and stir through, serve while hot.
9. ENJOY!

## *Easy noodle soup*

*Noodles, garlic, ginger, broth...what's not to love? I like to eat this when I feel like I am coming down with a cold, and for some reason, it seems to help! It's probably all in my head, but it seems to be a very health-inducing dish.*

**Serves:** 4-6 (4 large servings, 6 small servings)
**Time:** approximately 10 minutes

**Ingredients:**
- 5 blocks of dried ramen, (single serve blocks, about 1lb in total)
- 4 garlic cloves, crushed
- 1 tbsp grated fresh ginger
- 1 ¾ liters chicken stock
- 1 green onion, finely chopped

**Method:**
1. Press the FISH/VEGE/STEAM button on your PPC-XL and add a drizzle of oil.
2. Add the garlic and ginger and heat for about 20 seconds.
3. Add the stock and ramen, and secure the lid onto the pot.
4. Adjust the time to 4 minutes.
5. Once the pot beeps, carefully release the steam and remove the lid.
6. Stir the soup and serve in bowls.
7. Sprinkle the spring onion on top.
8. ENJOY!

### *Pressure cooker sausage stew*

*I like to buy my sausages from the butcher. They are usually far cheaper than at the supermarket, and they are made by the butcher with premium ingredients and no "filler" stuff. This stew is delicious and very moreish! The tomatoes add a hit of fresh sweetness, and the paprika brings a subtle smokiness.*

**Serves:** 6
**Time:** approximately 40 minutes

**Ingredients:**
- 5 sausages, chopped into 5 pieces each
- 1 onion, finely chopped
- 2 tins chopped tomatoes
- 1 beef stock cube and 1 ½ cups water
- 1 tsp paprika

**Method:**
1. Press the SOUP/STEW button on your PPC-XL and add a drizzle of oil.
2. Add the onion to the pot and sauté until soft.
3. Add the sausage pieces to the pot and sauté for a few minutes until browned.
4. Add the tomatoes, stock cube, water, paprika, salt, and pepper.
5. Secure the lid onto the pot and make sure the steam valve is closed.
6. Adjust the time to 30 minutes.
7. Once the pot beeps, carefully release the steam and remove the lid.
8. Stir the stew and serve hot.
9. ENJOY!

## *Minced lamb and tomato "stili" (stew and chili)*

*I call this "stili" because to me, it is a combination of a stew and a chili. You can use any kind of minced meat you like, but I enjoy using minced lamb as it gives a different flavor than the usual beef. You can eat this on its own, or use as a base for nachos or spaghetti!*

**Serves:** 6
**Time:** approximately 45 minutes

**Ingredients:**
- 3 lb minced lamb
- 1 onion, finely chopped
- 500ml lamb or beef stock
- 2 tins chopped tomatoes
- 1 tsp dried red chili, or chopped fresh red chili

**Method:**
1. Press the SOUP/STEW button on your PPC-XL and add a drizzle of oil.
2. Add the onion and chili and sauté until the onion is soft.
3. Add the lamb mince and sauté for a few minutes until browned.
4. Add the stock, tomatoes, salt, and pepper.
5. Secure the lid onto the pot and make sure the steam valve is closed.
6. Adjust the time to 30 minutes.
7. Once the pot beeps, carefully release the steam and remove the lid.
8. Stir the "stili" and serve while hot.
9. ENJOY!

## *Ham hock soup*

*It took me a long time to cotton on to the magic of ham hocks! Throw it in the PPC-XL with some water, veggies, seasoning...leave it to slow cook...and you'll be amazed at the outcome! Give it a go next time you feel like something easy, warming, and nourishing.*

**Serves:** 6
**Time:** approximately 2 hours and 15 minutes

**Ingredients:**
- 1 ham hock (flesh on)
- 1 onion, finely chopped
- 3 carrots, peeled and chopped into chunks
- 2 large potatoes, peeled and chopped into chunks
- 1 tin white beans

**Method:**
1. Press the SLOW COOK button on your PPC-XL and drizzle some oil into the pot.
2. Add the onion and sauté until soft.
3. Add the carrots, potatoes, beans, salt, and pepper to the pot and stir.
4. Place the ham hock into the pot and nestle it into the veggies.
5. Pour enough water into the pot to almost cover the ham hock.
6. Secure the lid onto the pot and keep the time at the default 2 hours.
7. Once the pot beeps, carefully release the steam and remove the lid.
8. Take the ham hock out of the pot and remove all of the meat from the bone.
9. Before you put the meat back into the pot, take a hand-held stick blender and blend the soup until it is mostly smooth but still has some chunks remaining.
10. Return the ham meat to the pot and stir through.
11. Serve while hot.
12. ENJOY!

## *Pork and apple stew*

Fruit in a stew?! Yes! Pork and apple are a match made in heaven. I use the slow cook function for this recipe as it ensures soft, pull-apart pork.

**Serves:** 6
**Time:** approximately 6 hours and 15 minutes

**Ingredients:**
- 4 lb pork shoulder (boneless), cut into large chunks tossed in flour
- 4 apples, cut into 6 pieces each
- 1 onion, finely chopped
- 1 ½ liters chicken stock
- 1 tsp mixed dried herbs (oregano, sage, rosemary…anything you've got!)

**Method:**
1. Press the SLOW COOK button on your PPC-XL and drizzle some oil into the pot.
2. Add the onion to the pot and sauté until soft.
3. Add the floured pork to the pot and cook for a few minutes until browned.
4. Add the apples, stock, herbs, salt, and pepper to the pot.
5. Secure the lid onto the pot and adjust the time to 6 hours.
6. Once the pot beeps, carefully release the steam and remove the lid.
7. Stir the stew, (the apples will break apart and release their sweetness throughout the dish).
8. Serve while hot.
9. ENJOY!

## *Beef and onion stew with wine*

*When red wine is reduced through cooking, the rich flavor is undeniably yummy. This recipe combines the deep flavors of red wine, onion, and beef. Serve with a side of buttery mashed potatoes.*

**Serves:** 6
**Time:** approximately 6 hours and 15 minutes

**Ingredients:**
- 4 lb stewing beef (chuck works really well), cut into chunks and tossed in flour
- 2 onions, roughly chopped
- 3 large potatoes, peeled and chopped into chunks
- 750ml red wine
- 500ml beef stock

**Method:**
1. Press the SLOW COOK button on your PPC-XL and drizzle some oil into the pot.
2. Add the onion to the pot and sauté until soft.
3. Add the floured beef to the pot and sauté for a few minutes until browned.
4. Add the potatoes, wine, beef stock, salt, and pepper.
5. Secure the lid onto the pot and adjust the time to 6 hours.
6. Once the pot beeps, release the steam and remove the lid.
7. Stir the stew and serve while hot.
8. ENJOY!

## Vegan and Vegetarian

Vegan and vegetarian diets are packed full of vital nutrients, minerals, and vitamins. We could all take a leaf from the book of a dedicated vegan or vegetarian! So, even if you are a die-hard meat eater, I encourage you to give these recipes a go. I promise you, you won't even be thinking about meat once you sink your teeth into these fabulous flavors!

## *Vegetarian chili (V, VG)*

*Beans, tomatoes, and spices come together to create this ultimate vegetarian chili. Serve it with nachos, on a baked potato, or alone with a dollop of Greek yoghurt and a side salad for a healthy and filling meal.*

**Serves:** 8 (yup, it makes a big batch! You can freeze any leftovers)
**Time:** approximately 45 minutes

## Ingredients:
- 4 tins beans, (approximately 3lb. Use a mixture of black and kidney, or all kidney)
- 2 tins chopped tomatoes (approximately 2lb)
- 2 onions, finely chopped
- 2 tsp paprika
- 2 tsp mixed spices: chili, cumin, coriander – use any dried savory spices you have, and adjust the amounts of chili powder to your spice preference

## Method:
1. Press the BEANS/LENTILS button on your PPC-XL and drizzle some oil into the pot.
2. Add the onions and sauté until soft.
3. Add the beans, tomatoes, paprika, and spices.
4. Secure the lid onto the pot and make sure the steam valve is closed.
5. Adjust the time to 30 minutes.
6. Once the pot beeps, carefully release the steam and remove the lid.
7. Stir a pinch of salt and people into the chili.
8. Serve while hot, with any dish you like, or on its own.
9. ENJOY!

## *Vegetarian fried rice (V)*

*Fried rice is one of those dishes that just hits the spot when you feel like something with carbs, a bit of saltiness, and a fresh punch of veggies. This recipe is super easy and delicious, and it's a great way to use up frozen veggies.*

**Serves:** 6
**Time:** 15 minutes

**Ingredients:**
- 2 ½ cups white rice
- 2 cups frozen vegetables, (I use the peas, corn, and carrot mixture)
- 3 eggs, lightly beaten
- 3 tbsp soy sauce
- 1 green onion, finely chopped

**Method:**
1. Press the RICE/RISOTTO button on your PPC-XL and make sure the time is at the 6-minute setting.
2. Rinse the rice and put it in your PPC-XL, add 2 ½ cups water and a pinch of salt.
3. Secure the lid onto the pot and make sure the steam valve is closed.
4. Once the pot beeps, carefully release the steam and remove the lid.
5. Take the rice out of the pot and set aside.
6. Keep the RICE/RISOTTO function on, and keep the lid off.
7. Drizzle some oil into the pot and once hot, add the vegetables and spring onions, sauté for a few minutes until cooked through.
8. Add the rice to the pot and combine with the vegetables.
9. Move the rice and vegetables to one side and add the eggs to the pot, lightly scrambling them as they cook.
10. Combine the lightly scrambled eggs with the rice.
11. Add the soy sauce and stir through.
12. Serve while hot with any extras such as hot sauce.
13. ENJOY!

## *Ginger, garlic, and honey tofu (V)*

*Tofu is sold at every supermarket, and it's a great ingredient to bulk-out a dish. Tofu is an amazing "flavor carrier" and this recipe calls on the gorgeous flavors of ginger, garlic, and honey. I like to use hard tofu, as opposed to the soft type.*

**Serves:** 4
**Time:** approximately 40 mins

**Ingredients:**
- 300g firm tofu, cut into strips (about 1cm thick)
- 1 tbsp fresh ginger, grated
- 4 garlic cloves, finely chopped
- 2 tbsp honey
- 1 tbsp soy sauce

**Method:**
1. In a small bowl, combine the ginger, garlic, honey, and soy sauce.
2. Place the tofu into the bowl and coat the tofu in the marinade, leave to sit for about 30 minutes.
3. Press the MEAT/CHICKEN button on your PPC-XL and drizzle some oil into the pot.
4. Once the oil is hot, add the tofu to the pot with the marinade.
5. Fry each piece of tofu on both sides until both sides are golden brown.
6. Serve as a side dish, or with some steamed vegetables.
7. ENJOY!

## *Sweet potato salad (V)*

*Fresh orange juice and red onion team up with sweet potato in this delicious salad. This salad is great warm and cold, so you can pack it into an airtight container and have it as a nutritious and delicious lunch.*

**Serves:** 6
**Time:** approximately 20 minutes

**Ingredients:**
- 4 lb sweet potato, skin on, chopped into chunks
- ½ large red onion, finely chopped
- Juice of 1 fresh orange
- 3 tbsp olive oil
- Fresh parsley, finely chopped

**Method:**
1. Pour 1 cup of water into the PPC-XL and place the steaming basket into the pot.
2. Place the sweet potatoes into the steaming basket and secure the lid onto the pot, make sure the steam valve is closed.
3. Press the FISH/VEG/STEAM button and adjust the time to 10 minutes.
4. Once the pot beeps, carefully release the steam and remove the lid.
5. Remove the sweet potato and put into a large bowl.
6. Add the red onion to the bowl with the sweet potatoes.
7. In a small bowl or cup, mix together the orange juice, olive oil, parsley, salt, and pepper to make a dressing.
8. Pour the dressing over the sweet potatoes and mix together until all combined and coated.
9. Serve warm or cold.
10. ENJOY!

## *Couscous, carrot, and seed salad (V)*

*If you're not used to using couscous, give it a go! I assure you, it's easy to prepare and yummy to eat. Carrot makes another appearance in this recipe, along with mixed seeds and honey.*

**Serves:** 6
**Time:** approximately 15 minutes

**Ingredients:**
- 2 cups couscous
- 3 carrots, peeled and cut into small chunks
- ¼ cup mixed seeds, (pumpkin and sunflower are the best choices)
- 1 tbsp honey
- 2 garlic cloves, crushed

**Method:**
1. Place couscous into a bowl and sprinkle it with salt and pepper.
2. Pour 2 ¼ cups boiling water over the couscous, stir, and then cover with a lid or with plastic wrap, leave to one side.
3. Press the MEAT/CHICKEN button on your PPC-XL and drizzle some oil into the pot.
4. Once the oil is hot, add the honey, garlic, and carrots. Sauté until the carrots are slightly caramelized and soft.
5. Add the seeds to the pot and toast them in the honey and oil for a minute or two.
6. Remove the lid or plastic from the couscous bowl, add a drizzle of olive oil, and "fluff" the couscous with a fork.
7. Add the carrot and seed mixture to the couscous and stir through until combined.
8. Serve warm or cold.
9. ENJOY!

## *Spinach risotto (V)*

*Risotto is one of those dishes that seems so impressive, despite being so easy to prepare. Well, the Power Pressure Cooker XL makes it easier than ever! This recipe uses spinach to add a pop of color and a touch of freshness.*

**Serves:** 4 – 6 (4 large servings, 6 smaller servings)
**Time:** approximately 15 minutes

### Ingredients:
- 2 cups risotto rice, (it's called Arborio rice and you can find it in the rice aisle at the supermarket)
- 4 cups vegetable stock
- 1 cup dry white wine
- 1 cup grated parmesan cheese
- 2 handfuls baby spinach leaves

### Method:
1. Press the RICE/RISOTTO button on your PPC-XL and manually adjust the time to 10 minutes.
2. Drizzle some olive oil into the pot and heat.
3. Add the rice to the pot and stir until coated in oil.
4. Add the wine and stir while it heats, until the wine has evaporated and soaked into the rice.
5. Add the stock and a sprinkle of salt and pepper.
6. Secure the lid onto the pot and make sure the steam valve is closed.
7. Once the pot beeps, carefully release the steam and remove the lid.
8. Add the spinach to the hot risotto and stir through until it wilts.
9. Add the Parmesan cheese and stir through until melted.
10. Serve while hot, with a sprinkling of fresh parsley.
11. ENJOY!

## *Spiced lentil soup (V, VG)*

*Lentils are one of the most affordable and easy-to-use ingredients. You can store dried lentils in your pantry to pull out when you are stuck for an idea for dinner. This lentil soup is warming, spicy, and very tasty indeed.*

**Serves:** 6
**Time:** approximately 35 minutes

**Ingredients:**
- 2 cups dried orange lentils
- 1 large onion, finely chopped
- 2 liters vegetable stock
- 1 tin chopped tomatoes
- 3 tsp mixed dried spices (I use an even amount of dried cumin, coriander, chili, cinnamon, garam masala…use what you've got!)

**Method:**
1. Press the BEANS/LENTILS button on your PPC-XL and adjust the time to 30 minutes.
2. Drizzle some oil into the pot and once warm, add the onion and spices, sauté until the onion is soft.
3. Add the lentils and stir until coated in spices.
4. Add the stock, tomatoes, and a sprinkling of salt and pepper, stir to combine.
5. Secure the lid onto the pot and make sure the steam valve is closed.
6. Once the pot beeps, carefully release the steam and remove the lid.
7. Stir the soup and serve while hot with a dollop of coconut cream and some fresh herbs.
8. ENJOY!

## Creamy vegetable curry (V, VG)

*If you don't have the vegetables listed in this recipe, use any other vegetables you have! The great thing about curry is that pretty much all vegetables work really well. Choose a red curry paste from the international section of your supermarket.*

**Serves:** 6
**Time:** approximately 20 minutes

**Ingredients:**
- 2 large potatoes, washed and cut into chunks
- 3 large carrots, cut into chunks
- 3 zucchinis, cut into chunks
- 3 tbsp red curry paste
- 2 cans coconut cream (about 900ml more or less)

**Method:**
1. Press the SOUP/STEW button on your PPC-XL and keep the time at the default 10 minutes.
2. Drizzle some oil into the pot and heat until warm.
3. Add the red curry paste and heat for about 1 minute.
4. Add the vegetables and stir until coated in curry paste.
5. Add the coconut cream, and 2 cups of water.
6. Secure the lid onto the pot and make sure the steam valve is closed.
7. Once the pot beeps, carefully release the steam and remove the lid.
8. Stir the curry and add a sprinkling of salt and pepper before serving.
9. Serve with white rice.
10. ENJOY!

## *Avocado and capsicum sushi (VG, V)*

*Sushi is far easier to make than you might think. I love to make sushi when I feel like a light dinner and a quick lunch the next day. This recipe uses creamy avocado and crunchy capsicum. You can add any other veggies you like, such as carrot, lettuce, and cucumber.*

**Serves:** makes 6 sushi rolls (about 36 pieces once cut)
**Time:** approximately 25 minutes

**Ingredients:**
- 6 nori sheets, (dried seaweed sheets)
- 1 ½ cups sushi rice, (or use brown rice and cook according to PPC-XL directions)
- 1 large avocado, flesh cut into strips
- 1 red capsicum, cut into strips
- Soy sauce

**Method:**
1. Press the RICE/RISOTTO button on your PPC-XL and adjust the time to 6 minutes (white rice).
2. Pour the rice into the pot and cover with 3 cups of water.
3. Secure the lid onto the pot and make sure the steam valve is closed.
4. Once the pot beeps, carefully release the steam and remove the lid, leave the rice to cool for about 30 minutes.
5. Lay the nori sheets onto a sushi mat, or onto a chopping board if you have no mat.
6. Spread a thin layer of rice over the nori sheet, leaving a 2-inch gap at the top.
7. Place avocado and capsicum in a line in the middle of the sheet, on top of the rice.
8. Tightly roll the sushi and seal the edge with some warm water.
9. Once all the rice, avocado, and capsicum have been used, slice the sushi rolls into approximately 6 pieces each.
10. Serve with soy sauce for dipping.
11. ENJOY!

### *Brown rice, cashew, and broccoli salad (VG, V)*

*Brown rice is nutty, chewy, and very nutritious. This salad features cashew nuts and broccoli, which come together to form a satisfying and filling salad for lunch or dinner.*

**Serves:** 6
**Time:** approximately 30 minutes

**Ingredients:**
- 2 cups brown rice
- ½ cup roasted and salted cashew nuts
- ½ a head of broccoli, cut into florets
- 2 garlic cloves, crushed
- 1 lemon

**Method:**
1. Press the RICE/RISOTTO button on your PPC-XL and adjust the time to 18 minutes (brown rice setting).
2. Add the rice to the pot and pour over 5 cups of water.
3. With a zester or fine grater, grate the zest of ½ a lemon into the pot.
4. Secure the lid onto the pot and make sure the steam valve is closed.
5. Once the pot beeps, carefully release the steam and remove the lid.
6. Remove the rice from the pot and set aside.
7. Rinse the pot out and place back into the PPC-XL.
8. Press the MEAT/CHICKEN button and drizzle some oil into the pot.
9. Once the oil is warm, add the garlic and sauté for about 30 seconds.
10. Add the broccoli florets and the zest of the second half of the lemon, sprinkle some salt and pepper over.
11. Sauté until the broccoli is beginning to become soft, but still has a crunchy bite.
12. Remove the broccoli and add to the bowl of rice, add the cashews.
13. Drizzle over some olive oil, and squeeze the juice from the lemon over the salad, stir to combine.
14. Serve warm or cold.
15. ENJOY!

## *Vegetarian burger patties (V, VG)*

*These vegetarian and vegan burger patties are full of nutrition and taste. I like to add beetroot slices and some feta cheese to my burgers when using these patties. You can add any toppings and condiments you desire!*

**Serves:** makes 8 patties
**Time:** approximately 25 minutes

### Ingredients:
- 2 tins chickpeas
- 1 onion, finely chopped
- 1 egg
- ½ cup breadcrumbs, (use old bread and pulse in the food processor if you don't have ready-made breadcrumbs)
- 1 tsp dried coriander, cumin, chili, or a mix of all 3

### Method:
1. Press the MEAT/CHICKEN button on your PPC-XL and drizzle some oil into the pot.
2. Add the onion and spices, sauté until the onion is soft.
3. Add the chickpeas and stir, sauté for a couple of minutes until the chickpeas are soft and beginning to crumble.
4. Remove the chickpea mixture from the pot, place into a bowl, and leave to cool slightly.
5. Add the egg, breadcrumbs, salt, and pepper to the bowl and combine with your hands or a wooden spoon until combined.
6. Drizzle some more oil into the pot and shape the mixture into round patties.
7. Fry the patties on both sides until golden (using the MEAT/CHICKEN function).
8. Assemble your burgers using your favorite ingredients.
9. ENJOY!

## *Olive and tomato spaghetti (V, VG)*

*This one-pot wonder can be called on when you've run out of fresh veggies, as all of the ingredients can be found in the pantry or lurking in the back of the fridge (olives!).*

**Serves:** 5
**Time:** approximately 20 minutes

**Ingredients:**
- 500g dried spaghetti
- 4 garlic cloves, finely chopped
- 2 tins chopped tomatoes
- ½ cup chopped black olives
- 1 tsp dried basil

**Method:**
1. Press the RICE/RISOTTO button and drizzle some oil into the pot.
2. Add the garlic to the pot and sauté for about 30 seconds.
3. Add the spaghetti, basil, olives, tomatoes, salt and pepper.
4. Add 2 cups of water, or enough so the pasta is just covered.
5. Adjust the time for 6 minutes, (white rice setting).
6. Secure the lid onto the pot and make sure the steam valve is closed.
7. Once the pot beeps, carefully release the steam and remove the lid.
8. Stir the pasta and sauce together.
9. Serve while hot.
10. ENJOY!

## *Lemon, pea, and parmesan penne pasta (V)*

Yes, another pasta dish! Lemon, peas, and parmesan create a fresh and vibrant flavor profile. This dish is just as delicious the next day, so make some extra to have as an easy lunch. For a vegan option, simply omit the parmesan.

**Servings:** 6
**Time:** approximately 20 minutes

**Ingredients:**
- 500gm dried penne pasta
- 3 garlic cloves, crushed
- 1 lemon
- 2 cups frozen peas
- ½ cup finely grated parmesan

**Method:**
1. Press the RICE/RISOTTO button on your PPC-XL and set the timer to 6 minutes, (white rice setting).
2. Drizzle some oil into the pot.
3. Add the garlic to the warm oil and sauté for about 30 seconds.
4. Finely grate the zest of half the lemon into the pot.
5. Add the peas, penne, salt, and pepper to the pot and cover with 2 cups of water, or enough to just cover the pasta.
6. Secure the lid onto the pot and make sure the steam valve is closed.
7. Once the pot beeps, carefully release the steam and remove the lid.
8. If there is excess water, simply drain it off; it doesn't matter if some of the garlic and lemon gets discarded, as the flavors will already have infused into the pasta and peas.
9. Drizzle with some olive oil, sprinkle the Parmesan on top, stir through, and serve while hot.
10. ENJOY!

## *Refried beans (V, VG)*

*This is more of a side dish than a main, and it's great for Mexican dinners. Tinned pinto beans are easy to find at the supermarket, and are really affordable. However, if you can't find pinto beans, simply use red kidney beans instead. Use as much chili powder as you like, according to your spice preference.*

**Serves:** makes 1 large bowl, about 5 servings
**Time:** approximately 20 minutes

**Ingredients:**
- 2 tins pinto beans, drained and rinsed
- 1 onion, finely chopped
- 2 tsp paprika
- 1 tsp chili powder, (more or less depending on preference)
- 1 tsp cumin

**Method:**
1. Press the BEANS/LENTILS button on your PPC-XL and drizzle some oil into the pot.
2. Add the onion to the warm oil and sauté until soft.
3. Add the beans, paprika, chili, and cumin to the pot and stir to combine.
4. Add ½ cup water to the pot with some salt and pepper, stir to combine.
5. Secure the lid onto the pot and make sure the steam valve is closed.
6. Adjust the time for 6 minutes.
7. Once the pot beeps, carefully release the steam and remove the lid, stir the beans.
8. Press the BEANS/LENTILS button again and sauté the bean mixture until very thick and mushy (you can use your spoon to mush the beans).
9. Serve however you like, (I like to serve with nachos).
10. ENJOY!

## *Crispy eggplant dippers (V)*

*I don't know about you, but I feel that eggplant is a totally under-utilized vegetable! Or maybe it's just me? Either way, I found a way of incorporating eggplant into my meals in the form of a starter. I like to call these "dippers" as you can dip them into any sauce or condiment.*

**Serves:** 4 – 6 as a starter
**Time:** approximately 15 minutes

**Ingredients:**
- 2 eggplants, cut into thick wedges
- 2 eggs, lightly beaten
- 1 cup fine bread crumbs mixed with ¼ cup flour

**Method:**
1. Press the MEAT/CHICKEN button on your PPC-XL and pour about ¼ cup oil into the pot.
2. On a large plate, mix together the bread crumbs, flour, salt, and pepper.
3. Dunk each eggplant wedge in the beaten egg and transfer to the plate of breadcrumbs to coat.
4. Once the oil in the pot is hot, fry the eggplant wedges in batches until each side is golden and crispy.
5. Transfer the fried wedges onto a plate lined with paper towels.
6. Serve with any sauce you like, (I like lemon mayonnaise and hot sauce).
7. ENJOY!

## *Rice noodles with cucumber, carrot, and sesame seeds (VG, V)*

*This is a fresh, Summery dish which can be eaten as a main or as a side dish during a multi-course meal. If you can't find limes, simply use lemons!*

**Serves:** 4 – 6 (4 servings as a main, 6 as a side dish)
**Time:** approximately 20 minutes

### Ingredients:
- 400g rice noodles, (I use the thicker, flatter kind of noodles, but you can use vermicelli if you like them to be thinner)
- ½ cucumber, peeled into strips with a potato peeler (lengthways)
- 2 carrots, peeled into strips with a potato peeler (lengthways)
- 2 tbsp sesame seeds, lightly toasted
- 1 lime (or lemon)

### Method:
1. Press the RICE/RISOTTO button on your PPC-XL and adjust the time to 3 minutes.
2. Place the rice noodles into the pot and pour over enough hot water to just cover the noodles.
3. Secure the lid onto the pot and make sure the steam valve is closed.
4. Once the pot beeps, carefully release the steam and remove the lid.
5. Drain the noodles and run them under some cold water to cool them down, place the noodles into a large bowl.
6. Drizzle the noodles with some oil, (use sesame oil if you have it).
7. Add the carrot, cucumber, sesame seeds, salt, pepper, and juice of the lime or lemon, stir to combine.
8. Serve alone or with other dishes.
9. ENJOY!

## *Pumpkin, peanut, and coconut side dish (VG, V)*

*I absolutely adore this side dish. You get the sweetness of the pumpkin, creaminess of the coconut, and saltiness of the peanuts...amazing. If you want to, you could eat this as a main dish, but because it's so full of rich flavor, I like to have it on the side of a lighter main meal.*

**Serves:** 6 (as a side dish)
**Time:** approximately 25 minutes

**Ingredients:**
- 500g pumpkin, skin removed, cut into chunks
- 4 garlic cloves, crushed
- 1 can coconut cream (about 400ml)
- 1/3 cup roasted, salted peanuts
- Fresh cilantro, finely chopped

**Method:**
1. Press the FISH/VEG/STEAM button on the PPC-XL and pour 1 cup of water into the pot.
2. Place the steaming basket into the pot and place the pumpkin chunks into the basket, sprinkle with salt.
3. Secure the lid onto the pot and make sure the steam valve is closed.
4. Once the pot beeps, carefully release the steam and remove the lid.
5. Take the pumpkin out of the pot and set aside, discard any excess water from the pot.
6. Press the MEAT/CHICKEN button and drizzle some oil into the pot.
7. Add the garlic to the pot and sauté for about 30 seconds.
8. Add the pumpkin and coconut cream to the pot and keep an eye on it while it sautés and the coconut cream becomes very thick.
9. Remove the pumpkin dish from the pot and sprinkle the peanuts and coriander over the top before serving.
10. ENJOY!

# Meat

If you are a meat-eater, you will love these recipes. I have included a mixture of beef, lamb, chicken and pork. There are simple recipes such as 'Roast chicken', which can be used as the base of a meal. There are also some recipes for more comprehensive and complete meals such as 'Rare steak strips with buttered corn'. It's always worth asking your butcher for the best cut of meat for the recipe at hand, as they can direct you to the best, (and often cheapest!) cuts.

## *Roast chicken*

*Roast chicken really needs no introduction! You could make this a day in advance for next-day chicken buns for lunch, or you could serve it straight from the pot with a pile of roasted potatoes and sweet peas...whatever your heart desires.*

**Serves:** makes 1 roast chicken
**Time:** approximately 50 minutes

**Ingredients:**
- 1 whole chicken, (small to medium sized)
- 1 lemon
- 1tbsp dried rosemary
- 1 cup water or chicken stock

**Method:**
1. Press the MEAT/CHICKEN button on your PPC-XL.
2. Drizzle some olive oil into the pot.
3. When the oil is hot, add the chicken to the pot (topside down) and brown the skin all over the bird, it will take about 3 minutes.
4. Remove the chicken from the pot and pour the water or stock into the bottom of the pot.
5. Place the steaming basket into the pot.
6. With a knife, poke holes into the lemon and place it inside the chicken cavity.
7. Generously season the chicken with salt, pepper, and dried rosemary by pressing it into the skin on top of the bird.
8. Place the chicken into the steaming basket and into the PPC-XL.
9. Secure the lid onto the pot and make sure the steam valve is closed, adjust the time to 40 minutes.
10. Once the pot beeps, carefully release the steam and remove the lid.
11. Take the chicken out of the pot and leave for 10 minutes to rest before carving.
12. ENJOY!

## *Roast beef*

*If you've got guests coming over, or want to serve your family something a bit special...go for an easy roast beef! Roast beef leftovers are great cold with a side salad, or even in a sandwich. Use any fresh herbs you have in the garden.*

**Serves:** makes a 3-4lb roast beef
**Time:** approximately 50 minutes

**Ingredients:**
- 3-4lb beef rump roast
- 1 onion, roughly chopped
- 1 liter beef stock
- Fresh herbs such as oregano, thyme and rosemary

**Method:**
1. Press the MEAT/CHICKEN button on your PPC-XL and adjust the time to 40 minutes.
2. Drizzle some oil into the pot.
3. Add the onions to the pot and sauté until soft.
4. Add the beef to the pot and sear until the entire surface has been browned, approximately 4 minutes.
5. Pour the stock into the pot and add the fresh herbs.
6. Secure the lid on the pot and make sure the steam valve is closed.
7. Once the pot beeps, carefully release the steam and remove the lid.
8. Remove the meat and leave it to rest.
9. Use the remaining onions and liquid in the pot to make an easy gravy by adding a spoonful of flour and more liquid to reach the desired consistency.
10. ENJOY!

## *Pork belly*

*Pork belly is a rich, sweet, and decadent meat. I like to serve it with freshly-steamed broccoli or a tangy slaw with vinegar dressing.*
*The Power Pressure Cooker XL makes pork belly a simple and easy meal to prepare.*

**Serves:** makes a 2lb pork belly, serves about 8-10
**Time:** approximately 50 minutes

**Ingredients:**
- 2 lb pork belly
- 2 cups stock, wine, or a mixture of both (vegetable or chicken stock is fine)
- 1 onion, roughly chopped
- Fresh herbs (any! Use your favorites)

**Method:**
1. Press the MEAT/CHICKEN button on your PPC-XL and adjust the time to 40 minutes.
2. Drizzle some oil into the pot.
3. Add the onions to the pot and sauté until soft.
4. Sprinkle the pork belly with a generous amount of salt and pepper, and rub it into the skin.
5. Place the pork belly into the pot and sear it on all sides until lightly browned, about 2 minutes.
6. Place the pork belly on top of the onions in the pot, (skin side up) and pour the wine/stock into the pot.
7. Secure the lid onto the pot and make sure the steam valve is closed.
8. Once the pot beeps, carefully release the steam and remove the lid.
9. Remove the pork from the pot and leave to rest while you use the remaining liquid to create a sauce or gravy.
10. ENJOY!

## *PPC-XL chili*

*Rich, spicy, meaty chili...feeling hungry yet? Serve with sour cream, guacamole, and tortilla chips, or on top of a baked potato with chives...the possibilities are endless!*

**Serves:** 6-8
**Time:** approximately 40 minutes

### Ingredients:
- 3 lb minced beef
- 2 tins kidney beans (about 800g), drained and rinsed
- 3 tins chopped tomatoes
- 1 onion, roughly chopped
- 4 tsp mixed savory spices, (paprika, chili powder, cumin, coriander)

### Method:
1. Press the SOUP/STEW button on your PPC-XL and adjust the time to 30 minutes.
2. Drizzle some oil into the pot.
3. Add the onions and sauté until soft.
4. Add the beef to the pot and cook for a few minutes until browned.
5. Add the beans, stock cube, tomatoes, spices, salt, pepper, and 1 cup water.
6. Secure the lid onto the pot and make sure the steam valve is closed.
7. Once the pot beeps, carefully release the steam and remove the lid.
8. Stir the chili and serve hot.
9. ENJOY!

## *Honey-glazed chicken drumsticks*

*Sweet, sticky chicken drumsticks remind me of Summertime dinners with fresh salads and crusty bread. They are just as yummy the next day, cold from the fridge.*

**Serves:** makes 8 drumsticks
**Time:** approximately 30 minutes

**Ingredients:**
- 8 chicken drumsticks
- 1 cup chicken stock or water
- 3 tbsp runny honey
- 1 tbsp soy sauce
- 1 tsp dried mixed herbs (etc. rosemary, oregano, thyme, tarragon, basil)

**Method:**
1. Press the MEAT/CHICKEN button on your PPC-XL and keep the time at the default 15 minutes.
2. In a large bowl, mix together honey, soy sauce, and herbs.
3. Coat each drumstick in the honey mixture and place them in the steaming basket (or onto a steaming rack).
4. Pour the stock into the bottom of the pot and place the steaming basket or rack (with the chicken inside) into the pot.
5. Secure the lid onto the pot and make sure the steam valve is closed.
6. Once the pot beeps, carefully release the steam and remove the lid.
7. Take the drumsticks out of the pot, sprinkle with salt and pepper, and leave to rest for 10 minutes before serving.
8. ENJOY!

## *Rare steak strips with buttered corn*

*Of course, if you like your steak well-done, then cook it to your liking. However, I prefer a blushing steak. This recipe pairs the succulent beef with sweet, buttery corn on the cob.*

**Serves:** 4
**Time:** approximately 20 minutes

**Ingredients:**
- 2 large beef steaks, (enough to be cut into 4 servings), I use eye fillet or rump
- 1 garlic clove, sliced in half, lengthways
- 1 tsp dried chili flakes
- 4 corn cobs
- 4 knobs of butter

**Method:**
1. Press the MEAT/CHICKEN button on your PPC-XL.
2. Rub the steaks with the cut side of the garlic clove.
3. Rub the steaks with a small amount of olive oil, and sprinkle the chili flakes over the top and gently press into the steak.
4. Once the pot is hot, cook the steaks for about 2 minutes on both sides until browned on the outside, but soft when pressed with your finger.
5. Remove the steaks from the pot and leave aside to rest.
6. Pour 1 cup of water into the pot (no need to rinse it out).
7. Press the FISH/VEG/STEAM button on the pot and keep the time at the default 2 minutes.
8. Place the steaming basket or rack into the pot and place the corn cobs on top.
9. Sprinkle the corn with salt.
10. Secure the lid onto the pot and make sure the steam valve is closed.
11. Once the pot beeps, carefully release the steam and remove the lid.
12. Take the corn out, place on a serving plate, and immediately rub each corn cob with butter.
13. Cut the steak into thin slices and serve with a buttered corn cob.
14. ENJOY!

## *Spicy coriander chicken*

*Chicken thighs are cheaper than chicken breasts, and they are much more flavorsome. Fresh coriander and red chili pack a major punch of flavor and heat with this easy and tasty recipe. Serve with brown rice and crunchy greens.*

**Serves:** makes 8 chicken thighs, (I suggest 1 or 2 thighs per serving)
**Time:** approximately 25 minutes

### Ingredients:
- 8 chicken thighs, boneless, skin on
- 1 onion, finely chopped
- 1 large handful fresh coriander, roughly chopped
- 1 fresh red chili, finely chopped
- 1 lime

### Method:
1. Press the MEAT/CHICKEN button on your PPC-XL and keep the time at the default 15 minutes, drizzle some oil into the pot.
2. Once the oil is hot, add the onion and sauté until soft.
3. In a large bowl, mix together the coriander, chili, and juice of 1 lime.
4. Add the chicken thighs to the bowl and toss until each thigh is covered in the coriander mixture.
5. Pour 1 cup of water into the bottom of the pot.
6. Place the coriander-coated chicken thighs into the steaming basket or rack and place into the pot.
7. Secure the lid onto the pot and make sure the steam valve is closed.
8. Once the pot beeps, carefully release the steam and remove the lid.
9. Remove the chicken from the pot and leave to rest for 10 minutes.
10. Use the leftover onions and liquid in the bottom of the pot to make a sauce or gravy if you wish.
11. ENJOY!

## *Pork and chive meatballs*

*This recipe uses minced pork, as I think it makes for a really amazing meatball. The chives give a gorgeous onion-y flavor. Serve with rich tomato sauce and spaghetti, or alone with a dipping sauce made from vinegar and soy sauce.*

**Serves:** 6 – 8
**Time:** approximately 25 minutes

**Ingredients:**
- 2 lb minced pork
- 1 egg
- ½ cup breadcrumbs
- ½ cup finely chopped chives

**Method:**
1. Press the MEAT/CHICKEN button on your PPC-XL and drizzle some oil into the pot, (a good amount, about 3tbsp).
2. Mix together the minced pork, egg, breadcrumbs, chives, salt, and pepper in a large bowl.
3. Roll the mixture into balls and place them into the pot once the oil is hot.
4. Cook the meatballs in batches until golden brown and cooked through.
5. Serve with toothpicks and a simple dipping sauce, or with a rich tomato sauce and pasta.
6. ENJOY!

## *Slow cooked lamb leg*

*Cooked for 2 hours, the lamb leg emerges from the pot soft, tender, and delicious. There are countless ways to serve this dish, but I like to serve it with mashed sweet potatoes and crunchy broccoli.*

**Serves:** 8 – 10
**Time:** approximately 2.5 hours

**Ingredients:**
- 1 leg of lamb, bone in
- 1 large sprig of fresh rosemary, (or 1tbsp dried if you don't have fresh)
- 2tbsp balsamic vinegar
- 4 garlic cloves, sliced in half, lengthways
- 2 cups lamb or beef stock

**Method:**
1. Press the SLOW COOK button on your PPC-XL and keep the time at the default 2 hours, make sure the steam valve is OPEN.
2. Drizzle some oil into the pot and leave to heat.
3. Rub the lamb leg with the cut sides of the garlic.
4. Rub the lamb leg with olive oil and sprinkle with salt.
5. Once the oil is hot, add the lamb leg to the pot (top side down) and brown the lamb until all sides are lightly browned, (about 4 minutes of turning the lamb in the pot to sear).
6. Settle the lamb in the pot, (top side up) and pour the balsamic vinegar over the top.
7. Pour the stock into the pot and add the cut garlic cloves.
8. Secure the lid onto the pot and leave for 2 hours.
9. Once the pot beeps, carefully remove the lid and take the lamb out of the pot, leave to rest while you use the leftover liquid to make a sauce or gravy if you wish.
10. ENJOY!

## *Pork chops with lemon zest*

*Pork chops are a great mid-week dinner. This recipe uses the freshness of lemon zest which really lifts the flavor of the meat. I like to serve these pork chops with freshly-made apple sauce and of course...fresh greens!*

**Serves:** makes 6 pork chops
**Time:** approximately 25 minutes

**Ingredients:**
- 6 pork chops
- 1 lemon
- 1 onion, finely chopped
- 2 garlic cloves, crushed

**Method:**
1. Press the MEAT/CHICKEN button on your PPC-XL and keep the time to the default 15 minutes.
2. Drizzle some oil into the pot.
3. Season the pork chops with salt and pepper.
4. Once the oil is hot, sear each pork chop on both sides until brown.
5. Remove the pork chops from the pot and set aside.
6. Add the garlic and onion to the pot, sauté until the onion is soft.
7. With a zester or fine grater, grate the zest of the whole lemon into the pot, and squeeze the juice from the whole lemon into the pot also.
8. Pour ¼ cup water into the pot and stir to combine all ingredients.
9. Add the pork chops to the pot.
10. Secure the lid onto the pot and make sure the steam valve is closed.
11. When the pot beeps, carefully release the steam and remove the lid.
12. Remove the pork chops from the pot and leave to rest.
13. Stir the remaining mixture in the bottom of the pot and keep it to be spooned on top of the pork chops before serving.
14. ENJOY!

## *Crumbed chicken*

*I guess you could call this a "healthier version of fried chicken", in the sense that the outside of the chicken is crispy, and the inside is soft and juicy.*

**Serves:** makes 8 pieces
**Time:** approximately 25 minutes

**Ingredients:**
- 8 chicken thighs, drumsticks, or legs, (bone in, skin on)
- 2 eggs, lightly beaten
- ½ cup finely grated Parmesan
- 1 cup bread crumbs
- 1tsp garlic salt (or salt mixed with 1 clove crushed garlic if you don't have garlic salt)

**Method:**
1. Press the MEAT/CHICKEN button on your PPC-XL and pour about 4tbsp oil into the pot.
2. In a large bowl, mix together the Parmesan, bread crumbs, garlic salt, and pepper.
3. Dip each chicken piece into the beaten egg, then transfer straight to the breadcrumbs, and coat.
4. Once the oil is hot, cook the chicken in batches, turning every couple of minutes, so that each side of the chicken is crispy and golden.
5. Once all of the chicken has cooked through, (the juices are running clear and there is no pink flesh to be seen) leave to rest on a board for 10 minutes.
6. ENJOY!

## *Beef stir fry with garlic and soy*

*Dinner doesn't get much easier than this. Tender strips of beef, garlic, soy sauce, and fresh vegetables...throw it all in a bowl, and go for it! If you don't have the vegetables listed in this recipe, use whatever else you've got.*

**Serves:** 6
**Time:** approximately 20 minutes

**Ingredients:**
- 2 large steaks, (cheaper cuts are fine) sliced into thin strips
- 4 garlic cloves, crushed
- 2 large carrots, cut into thin strips
- 2 large zucchinis, cut into strips
- 2 tbsp soy sauce

**Method:**
1. Press the MEAT/CHICKEN button on your PPC-XL and drizzle some oil into the pot.
2. Once hot, add the beef and stir-fry for about 2 minutes or until slightly browned but not cooked through.
3. Add the carrot, zucchini, soy sauce, and garlic.
4. Stir-fry until the meat has reached your desired doneness and the vegetables are still crunchy to the bite.
5. Serve with rice, noodles, or on its own.
6. ENJOY!

## *Creamy lemon chicken*

*For this recipe, I find that boneless chicken breast or thigh works best. A great recipe to use if you've got an abundance of lemons. This can be served on its own with a side of vegetables, or with fettuccine, for a rich and decadent dinner.*

**Serves:** 6
**Time:** approximately 25 minutes

**Ingredients:**
- 4 chicken breasts, or 6 chicken thighs (chicken breast tends to be larger than thighs so 4 suffices for 6 people), cut into large chunks
- 2 lemons
- 1 cup heavy cream
- 1 cup chicken stock
- 1 tsp dried rosemary

**Method:**
1. Press the MEAT/CHICKEN button on your PPC-XL and leave the time at the default 15 minutes.
2. Drizzle some oil into the pot.
3. Once the oil is hot, add the chicken and sauté each side until golden brown.
4. With a zester or fine grater, grate the zest from one whole lemon into the pot.
5. Squeeze the juice from 2 lemons into the pot.
6. Add the cream, stock, rosemary, salt, and pepper to the pot and stir to combine.
7. Secure the lid onto the pot and make sure the steam valve is closed.
8. Once the pot beeps, carefully release the steam and remove the lid.
9. Give the mixture a stir, and remove the chicken.
10. If the sauce is still too runny, press the MEAT/CHICKEN button again, and simply simmer it until it reaches the desired thickness.
11. Pour the sauce over the chicken before serving.
12. ENJOY!

## *Sausage and potato bake*

*This is one of those dishes which is so comforting, yet so easy. Use any sausages you like; personally, I like to use sausages from the butcher, as they are fresh, well-made, and don't have as many additives as supermarket varieties. Lamb, pork, or beef sausages are ideal for this dish.*

**Serves:** 6
**Time:** approximately 40 minutes

**Ingredients:**
- 6 sausages
- 3 large potatoes, cut into small chunks
- 1 onion, roughly chopped
- ½ tin chopped tomatoes (about ¾ cup)

**Method:**
1. Press the MEAT/CHICKEN button on your PPC-XL and adjust the time to 30 minutes.
2. Drizzle some oil into the pot.
3. Add the onions and sauté until soft.
4. Add the potatoes and sauté with the onions for 5 minutes.
5. In a heatproof dish, (one that fits into the PPC-XL) place the sausages, potatoes, onion, and tomatoes.
6. Pour 1 cup of water into the bottom of the pot, and sit the dish inside the pot on a trivet.
7. Secure the lid onto the pot and make sure the steam valve is closed.
8. Once the pot beeps, carefully release the steam and remove the lid.
9. Remove the dish from the pot.
10. If you like, you can sprinkle some cheese on top and place the dish in the oven, under the grill until the cheese melts.
11. Or else, serve with a side of green veggies.
12. ENJOY!

## *Spicy pork rice bowl*

*This is a great dish for when you feel like a bit of starchy comfort, tasty meat, and a fuss-free preparation. You can use any type of rice you like, but I find sushi rice to be perfect for this dish.*

**Serves:** 4
**Time:** approximately 30 minutes

**Ingredients:**

- 4 pork steaks, (or 3 if the steaks are very big) cut into small pieces
- 1 red chili, finely chopped
- 3 tbsp soy sauce
- 2 tbsp white wine vinegar (or apple cider vinegar)
- 2 cups sushi rice

**Method:**

1. Press the RICE/RISOTTO button on your PPC-XL and keep the time at the default 6 minutes (white rice setting).
2. Add the rice to the bowl and enough water according to the instructions on your rice packet.
3. Secure the lid onto the pot and make sure the steam valve is closed.
4. In a bowl, mix together the chili, soy sauce, vinegar, and ¼ cup water.
5. Add the pork to the bowl and leave to marinade while the rice cooks.
6. Once the pot beeps, carefully release the steam and remove the lid.
7. Remove the rice from the pot and keep to one side, rinse out the pot.
8. Press the MEAT/CHICKEN button on your PPC-XL and keep the time at the default 15 minutes, drizzle some oil into the pot.
9. Once the oil is hot, add the pork and marinade to the pot and sauté for 1 minute to seal.
10. Secure the lid onto the pot and make sure the steam vent is closed.
11. Once the pot beeps, carefully release the steam and remove the lid.
12. Serve the pork on top of the rice, in a bowl, with an extra dash of soy sauce, and any other toppings you like, such as spring onions, shredded carrot, and freshly sliced cucumber.
13. ENJOY!

## *Beef and bean burger patties*

*Not just any old burger patties, these are packed-full of extra flavor with the help of black beans, spices, and soy sauce. Serve on a toasted sesame bun with a fresh coleslaw and lemon mayonnaise…yum.*

**Serves:** makes 8 patties
**Time:** approximately 25 minutes

**Ingredients:**
- 2 lb minced beef
- 1 tin black beans, drained and rinsed
- 1 egg
- 3 tsp mixed spices, (cumin, coriander, chili etc. use what you have and like)
- 3 tbsp soy sauce

**Method:**
1. In a large bowl, mix together the minced beef, beans, egg, spices, soy sauce, a small pinch of salt, and pepper until combined.
2. Press the MEAT/CHICKEN button on your PPC-Xl and drizzle about 3tbsp oil into the pot.
3. Shape the patty mixture into patties and cook them in batches, frying both sides for about 2 minutes each, or until they reach the desired doneness, and are golden brown on both sides.
4. Serve however you like!
5. ENJOY!

# Seafood

If you don't already include seafood into your diet, then start! (Unless you are vegan or vegetarian, of course!). Fish and seafood is full of skin and brain-loving treats such as fatty acids. My personal favorite fish is salmon, so you'll find a few salmon-based recipes here! There are also some amazing white fish, tuna, and prawn recipes. The PPC-XL makes cooking seafood a cinch, so get cookin'!

## *Simple sautéed sesame salmon*

*Just like the name suggests, this salmon recipe is simple yet delicious. Use fresh salmon if you can, and make sure to remove the bones if they haven't already been removed by the fishmonger. Black sesame seeds look very classy, but just use white seeds if you want!*

**Serves:** 4
**Time:** approximately 15 minutes

**Ingredients:**
- 4 salmon filets
- 4tbsp sesame seeds, mixture of black and white (or just white if you can't get black ones)

**Method:**
1. Press the MEAT/CHICKEN button on your PPC-XL and drizzle some oil into the pot.
2. On a plate, mix together 1tsp salt with the sesame seeds.
3. Rub the salmon fillets with a small amount of oil.
4. Roll each salmon fillet in the salt and sesame seeds until both sides are coated.
5. Sauté the salmon fillets in batches of 2 (or 1 if they are very large) for about 2 minutes each side.
6. Serve while hot, with your favorite vegetables.
7. ENJOY!

## *Crispy crumbed fish with lemon mayonnaise*

*Fish and lemon are like two peas in a pod, they go together SO well! Creamy, tangy mayonnaise is the perfect accompaniment to these crispy, light pieces of fish. Use any white fish you can find! Fresh is best.*

**Serves:** 6 as a light starter
**Time:** approximately 15 minutes

### Ingredients:
- 6 small fillets of white fish such as snapper or cod, cut in half, lengthways
- 2 eggs, lightly beaten
- 1 cup fine breadcrumbs, toasted in the oven until crispy but not burnt
- ½ cup good-quality mayonnaise
- 1 large lemon

### Method:
1. First, prepare the lemon mayonnaise by finely grating the zest of the whole lemon into the mayonnaise, then mix through the juice from the whole lemon into the mayonnaise. Add a sprinkle of pepper, and stir until all ingredients are combined. Done!
2. Press the MEAT/CHICKEN button on your PPC-XL and drizzle some oil into the pot.
3. Mix the breadcrumbs with salt and pepper, and spread out on a plate.
4. Dip each piece of fish into the beaten egg until coated.
5. Transfer the egg-coated fish to the breadcrumbs and thoroughly coat.
6. Cook the fish in batches in the hot oil, cooking both sides for about 2 minutes each, or until golden and crispy on the outside.
7. Serve the fish with the lemon mayonnaise on the side.
8. ENJOY!

## *White fish poached in tomato and olive sauce*

*Light, tender fish gets a makeover with the briny flavors of tinned tomatoes and black olives. A wonderful dish for a light meal. Pair with a glass of red wine. The same rule goes...use any fresh, white fish you can find! I like to use Snapper.*

**Serves:** 6
**Time:** approximately 20 minutes

**Ingredients:**
- 6 white fish fillets
- 4 garlic cloves, crushed
- 2 tins chopped tomatoes
- 1/3 cup chopped black olives
- ¼ cup dry white wine

**Method:**
1. Press the BEANS/LENTILS button on your PPC-XL keep the time at the default 5 minutes.
2. Drizzle some oil into the pot and add the garlic, sauté for about 30 seconds.
3. Add the white wine and cook for about 2 minutes until reduced.
4. Add the tomatoes, salt, and pepper, simmer for about 4 minutes until slightly reduced and thickened.
5. Stir the olives into the tomatoes.
6. Place the fish fillets on top of the tomato mixture and press down so they are almost submerged.
7. Secure the lid onto the pot and make sure the steam valve is closed.
8. Once the pot beeps, carefully release the steam and remove the lid.
9. Serve the fish with the tomato and olive sauce on top.
10. ENJOY!

## *Lemon prawn starter snacks*

*These lemony delights are fantastic as a classy starter for dinner parties or special dinners.*

**Serves:** about 6 as a small starter
**Time:** approximately 10 minutes

**Ingredients:**
- 3 lb prawns (tiger prawns are best)
- 3 garlic cloves, crushed
- 2 lemons

**Method:**
1. Press the MEAT/CHICKEN button on your PPC-XL and drizzle some oil into the pot.
2. Add the garlic and sauté for about 30 seconds.
3. Finely grate the zest from 1 whole lemon into the pot and squeeze the juice from both lemons into the pot.
4. Add the prawns to the pot and sprinkle over some salt and pepper.
5. Toss the prawns in the lemon and garlic and sauté until they turn pink.
6. Serve on a platter with toothpicks.
7. ENJOY!

## *Spicy prawn ramen*

*Ramen is having such a popular moment, and for good reason! Easy and affordable, these delicious noodles pair extremely well with prawns. This recipe adds simple flavors such as chili and soy to really lift the flavor profile.*

**Serves:** 4
**Time:** approximately 20 minutes

**Ingredients:**
- 4 blocks dried ramen
- 2lb prawns
- 4 garlic cloves, crushed
- 2tsp dried chili flakes
- 1tbsp soy sauce

**Method:**
1. Place the ramen blocks into a large bowl and pour over enough boiling water to cover them, place a lid or tight plastic wrap over the bowl and leave aside.
2. Press the MEAT/CHICKEN button on your PPC-XL and drizzle some oil into the pot.
3. Add the garlic and chili, sauté for 30 seconds.
4. Add the prawns, salt, and pepper, sauté until pink.
5. Drain the ramen and pour the cooked noodles into the PPC-XL with the prawns.
6. Add the soy sauce and toss through, combining the noodles, soy, and prawns together.
7. Serve while hot.
8. ENJOY!

## *Fish cakes with parsley*

*Fish cakes are lovely for a summertime lunch or light dinner. This recipe uses smoked fish for a deep flavor, and parsley for freshness.*

**Serves:** 6 (about 3 fish cakes each)
**Time:** approximately 35 minutes

**Ingredients:**
- 1lb smoked fish, flaked
- 1 egg, lightly beaten
- ¼ cup fresh parsley, chopped
- 2 large potatoes, peeled and chopped into chunks

**Method:**
1. Press the SOUP/STEW button on your PPC-XL and keep the time at the default 10 minutes, place the potatoes into the pot.
2. Add enough water to only just cover the potatoes, sprinkle some salt over the top.
3. Secure the lid onto the pot and make sure the steam valve is closed.
4. Once the pot beeps, carefully release the steam and remove the lid.
5. Drain the water from the pot and remove the potatoes, place them in a large bowl, leave to cool for 10 minutes.
6. Mash the potatoes with a masher and add the flaked fish, parsley, egg, salt, and pepper, stir until combined.
7. Press the MEAT/CHICKEN button on the PPC-XL and drizzle a generous amount of oil into the pot (about 3tbsp).
8. Once the oil is hot, shape the fish cake mixture into round patties, and cook in batches, turning once, until golden brown on each side.
9. Serve with any sauces and condiments you like.
10. ENJOY!

## *Fish stew*

*Simple as that...fish stew. Tomatoes, spices, fish, and onions all in one easy dish. Serve with crusty bread and butter and a glass of red...dinner is served!*

**Serves:** 6
**Time:** approximately 40 minutes

**Ingredients:**
- 2lb white fish, cut into chunks
- 1 large onion, finely chopped
- 3 tins chopped tomatoes
- 1 tsp paprika
- 2 tsp mixed spices (chili, cumin, coriander...whatever's on hand)

**Method:**
1. Press the SOUP/STEW button on your PPC-XL and adjust the time for 30 minutes, drizzle some oil into the pot.
2. Once the oil is hot, add the onion and sauté until soft.
3. Add the spices, and sauté with the onions for about 1 minute.
4. Add the tomatoes, salt, pepper, 1 cup of water, and stir to combine.
5. Add the fish and make sure the fish pieces are submerged in the tomatoes.
6. Secure the lid onto the pot and make sure the steam valve is closed.
7. Once the pot beeps, carefully release the steam and remove the lid.
8. Stir the stew and serve hot, with a sprinkling of fresh parsley.
9. ENJOY!

## *Fish with lemon and coconut rice*

*Coconut rice is such a gorgeous accompaniment to fish, and the lemon makes it even more delightful. You could use salmon instead of white fish if you wanted a richer-tasting dish.*

**Serves:** 4
**Time:** approximately 25 minutes

**Ingredients:**
- 4 fillets of fish, (any fish you like)
- 1 ripe lemon, cut into 8 slices
- 2 cups white rice
- 1 tin coconut milk (about 400ml)
- 1 cup water or fish stock

**Method:**
1. Press the RICE/RISOTTO button on your PPC-XL and keep the time to the default 6 minutes, (white rice setting).
2. Add the rice to the pot and pour the coconut milk and stock or water into the pot, add a pinch of salt, stir.
3. Secure the lid onto the pot and make sure the steam valve is closed.
4. Once the pot beeps, carefully release the steam and remove the lid.
5. Take the rice out of the pot and place in a bowl to the side.
6. Rinse the pot out, and press the MEAT/CHICKEN button, drizzle some oil into the pot.
7. Sprinkle the fish with salt and pepper and place 2 lemon slices on each fillet.
8. Once the oil is hot, cook the fish fillets in batches, until the bottom is golden brown and the fish is cooked through.
9. Serve each fillet of fish on a bed of coconut rice, with the lemon slices on the side to be squeezed over the fish before eating.
10. ENJOY!

### *Easy tuna and pea pasta*

*I turn to this recipe when the cupboards are looking a bit bare. I always have penne pasta and tins of tuna in the pantry, and frozen peas in the freezer. A sprinkle of grated Parmesan goes a long way if you have it! Otherwise, eat as it is, and you'll love it.*

**Serves:** 4
**Time:** approximately 20 minutes

**Ingredients:**
- 4 cups dried penne pasta
- 200g (approximately) tinned tuna (1 large tin, or 2 small tins)
- 1 ½ cup frozen peas
- 1 lemon
- ½ cup grated parmesan (if you have it, can use cheddar instead)

**Method:**
1. Press the RICE/RISOTTO button on your PPC-XL and keep the time at the default 6 minutes, (white rice setting).
2. Add the pasta, peas, zest of the lemon, salt, and pepper to the pot, cover with enough water to cover the pasta.
3. Secure the lid onto the pot and make sure the steam valve is closed.
4. Once the pot beeps, carefully release the steam and remove the lid, drain any excess water.
5. Add the tuna and cheese to the pot and stir through with a squeeze of lemon juice.
6. Serve with an extra sprinkling of cheese.
7. ENJOY!

## *Steamed scallops*

*It takes only a few minutes to create this decadent starter. Scallops are delicious, and this recipe enhances their lovely flavor with only a few simple ingredients.*

**Serves:** 4 as a starter, (3 each)
**Time:** approximately 7 minutes

**Ingredients:**
1. 12 scallops in shells
- 1 small red onion, finely chopped
- 30g butter, cut into small pieces
- 1 tbsp white wine vinegar

**Method:**
1. In a small bowl, combine onion, vinegar, salt, pepper, and 3tbsp olive oil.
2. Remove the scallops from their shells and keep one half of each shell.
3. Place the scallops back into one half of their shell, and spoon over a spoonful of onion/vinegar mixture.
4. Press the FISH/STEAM/VEG button on your PPC-XL and adjust the time to 4 minutes.
5. Pour 2 cups of water into the bottom of the pot and place the steaming basket into the pot.
6. Place the scallops into the basket (careful not to spill the onion sauce!).
7. Secure the lid onto the pot and make sure the steam valve is closed.
8. Once the pot beeps, carefully release the steam and remove the lid.
9. Remove the scallops from the steaming basket and place onto a serving plate, spoon over the remainder of the onion sauce before serving.
10. ENJOY!

## Crab macaroni

*Macaroni is a crowd favorite, and this recipe has been upgraded with the addition of crabmeat. This recipe doesn't use the usual cheese sauce, but instead uses grated cheese alone for a lighter dish.*

**Serves:** 4 – 6
**Time:** approximately 25 minutes

### Ingredients:
- 4 cups dried macaroni
- 1 onion, finely chopped
- 2 cups crab meat, chopped
- 2 cups grated cheddar cheese
- 1 cup heavy cream

### Method:
1. Cook the pasta according to the packet instructions, (use the PPC-XL to do this, or simply boil in a regular pot).
2. Press the MEAT/CHICKEN button on your PPC-XL and drizzle some oil into the pot.
3. Add the onion to the pot and sauté until soft.
4. Add the crab, cream, and cheese, stir until the cheese has melted and the mixture is thick.
5. Add the cooked macaroni and stir to combine.
6. Serve as is, or place in a dish and place under the grill in the oven with extra cheese on top.
7. ENJOY!

## *Golden rice with mixed seafood*

*The "golden" rice comes from the addition of turmeric. If you don't have turmeric, you can find it at any supermarket, in the dried spices section. This recipe uses mixed frozen seafood for a cheap and easy option.*

**Serves**: 6
**Time:** approximately 30 minutes

**Ingredients:**
- 2 cups white rice
- 1 tsp powdered turmeric
- 1 onion, finely chopped
- 3 cups mixed frozen seafood
- Fresh parsley, chopped

**Method:**
1. Press the RICE/RISOTTO and keep the time to the default 6 minutes, (white rice setting).
2. Place the rice, a pinch of salt, and turmeric into the pot and stir.
3. Pour 3 cups of water into the pot and stir.
4. Secure the lid onto the pot and make sure the steam valve is closed.
5. Once the pot beeps, carefully release the steam and remove the lid.
6. Remove the rice from the pot and place in a bowl to the side.
7. No need to wash the pot. Press the MEAT/CHICKEN button and add a drizzle of oil.
8. Add the onion to the pot and sauté until soft.
9. Add the seafood to the pot and sauté until pink and cooked through.
10. Serve the seafood on top of the golden rice, with a generous sprinkle of chopped fresh parsley.
11. ENJOY!

## *Mussels with garlic and wine*

All mussels need is a dash of white wine, a sprinkle of salt, and some freshly crushed garlic. Serve with fresh bread as a light lunch or starter.

**Serves:** 4
**Time:** approximately 15 minutes

**Ingredients:**
- 12 fresh mussels, in shells
- 4 garlic cloves, crushed
- ½ cup dry white wine

**Method:**
1. Press the MEAT/CHICKEN button on your PPC-XL and drizzle some oil into the pot.
2. Add the garlic wine, and salt, simmer until reduced.
3. Pour the wine and garlic sauce into a jug and set aside.
4. Press the FISH/VEG/STEAM button on your PPC-XL and adjust the time to 4 minutes, pour 2 cups of water into the pot (no need to rinse the pot).
5. Place the mussels in the steaming basket and place into the pot.
6. Secure the lid onto the pot and make sure the steam valve is closed.
7. Once the pot beeps, carefully release the steam and remove the lid.
8. Take the mussels out of the basket and place on a serving plate.
9. Open the shells wide and pour the wine sauce evenly over the mussels.
10. ENJOY!

## *Zesty cabbage and fish salad*

*Lemon juice, red cabbage, and fresh fish are a fabulous salad combination. The crunchy textures and fresh flavors are incredibly satisfying and moreish.*

**Serves:** 6
**Time:** approximately 15 minutes

**Ingredients:**
- 4 white fish fillets
- 1 red cabbage, very finely sliced
- 2 ripe lemons
- Large handful fresh coriander, finely chopped

**Method:**
1. Press the FISH/VEG/STEAM button on your PPC-XL and adjust the time to 4 minutes.
2. Place the fish fillets in the steaming basket and place in the pot, sprinkle the fish with salt and pepper.
3. Secure the lid onto the pot and make sure the steam valve is closed.
4. Once the pot beeps, carefully release the steam and remove the lid.
5. Take the fish out of the steaming basket and leave aside to cool.
6. In a large bowl, combine the red cabbage, juice of 2 lemons, 2tbsp olive oil, salt, and pepper.
7. Flake the fish fillets with a fork and stir through the cabbage salad.
8. Serve immediately.
9. ENJOY!

## *Hot, fresh salmon broth with Asian greens*

*This dish features clear broth, fresh salmon, and crunchy Asian greens. A perfect Winter dish, or for when you feel like something light and healthy, yet comforting.*

**Serves:** 4
**Time:** approximately 20 minutes

**Ingredients:**
- 2 liters fish stock
- 4 garlic cloves, crushed
- 2 tbsp soy sauce
- 2 large fresh salmon fillets, sliced into thin slices
- 2 large bunches Pak Choi or Bok Choy, base removed and leaves separated

**Method:**
1. Press the FISH/VEG/STEAM button on your PPC-XL and adjust the time to 2 minutes.
2. Place the fish stock, garlic, and soy sauce in the pot.
3. Place the steaming basket in the pot and place the Asian greens in the basket.
4. Secure the lid onto the pot, and make sure the steam valve is closed.
5. Once the pot beeps, carefully release the steam and remove the lid.
6. Remove the basket with the Asian greens inside, and set it to one side.
7. Immediately place the salmon slices in the pot, and submerge them in the hot fish stock, wait 2 minutes, (the salmon will cook in the hot stock, no extra heat required).
8. Stir the soy sauce through the stock and salmon and divide into bowls.
9. Place Asian greens on top of the salmon and broth, serve while hot.
10. ENJOY!

### *Mini fish tacos with minted yogurt*

*Fish tacos seem like a treat food, but in fact, these ones are super healthy! This recipe is just a guideline; you can add any ingredients you like, to create the ultimate fish taco just how you like it. You can use regular-sized taco shells, but I quite like the little ones.*

**Serves:** 4
**Time:** approximately 25 minutes

**Ingredients:**
- 12 mini soft taco shells/wraps
- 2 large white fish fillets
- ½ red cabbage, finely sliced
- ½ cup thick Greek yoghurt
- Fresh coriander, chopped

**Method:**
1. Press the MEAT/CHICKEN button on the PPC-XL and drizzle some oil into the pot.
2. Sprinkle the fish with salt, pepper, and any herbs or spices you'd like to use to enhance the flavor.
3. Fry the fish on both sides in the pot, until both sides are golden and the fish is cooked through.
4. Remove the fish from the pot and flake with a fork, or simply slice into small pieces.
5. With the pot still on, place the soft taco shells/wraps into the pot and heat for about 30 seconds each, (this is to heat the shells, and also to soak up some of the lovely fish-flavored oil from the bottom of the pot).
6. Assemble the tacos by placing a bed of cabbage onto each shell, then a generous amount of fish, then a dollop of Greek yoghurt, and finally, a generous sprinkling of fresh coriander.
7. Eat immediately.
8. ENJOY!

# Dessert

If you are anything like me, then you have a MAJOR sweet tooth. In case you didn't already know…you can make incredible desserts in your Power Pressure Cooker XL. Beware; it's so easy to create sweet treats in the PPC-XL you might find yourself indulging a little more often than you'd planned…

I have compiled a list of great desserts for all tastes. Lemons, berries, chocolate, caramel, cream, cheesecake and more star in this epic ending to our recipe section. Note: these recipes use grams as opposed to pounds as I find it makes for a better and more accurate measurement.

## *Chocolate pots*

*Rich, dark, velvety chocolate ...one of the best dessert flavors under the sun! Use good-quality dark chocolate, and serve with fresh, plump raspberries.*

**Serves:** 6
**Time:** approximately 30 minutes

### Ingredients:
- 300ml heavy cream
- 50ml full fat milk
- 200g dark chocolate
- 30g brown sugar
- 3 egg yolks

### Method:
1. In a medium bowl, whisk together the egg yolks and sugar until the sugar has dissolved and the mixture is pale.
2. Pour the cream and milk into a small bowl and place in the microwave for 20-second increments, until hot.
3. Break the chocolate up into small pieces and put it in the bowl with the milk and cream, stir until the chocolate has melted and the mixture is smooth and silky, leave aside until cool.
4. Pour the egg and sugar mixture into the chocolate mixture, whisking the whole time until combined.
5. Grease 6 ramekins with butter and fill with even amounts of mixture.
6. Press the FISH/VEGE/STEAM button on the PPC-XL and adjust the time to 10 minutes.
7. Pour 2 cups of water into the pot and place a trivet into the pot.
8. Place the ramekins on top of the trivet, secure the lid onto the pot, and make sure the steam valve is closed.
9. Once the pot beeps, carefully release the steam, remove the lid, take the ramekins out of the pot and leave to cool and set.
10. Serve with fresh raspberries.
11. ENJOY!

## *Caramelized bananas and ice cream*

*This recipe really couldn't be simpler. Soft, caramelized bananas on top of sweet, cold ice cream is a winning combination. Kids love this dessert just as much as grown-ups!*

**Serves:** 6
**Time:** approximately 10 minutes

**Ingredients:**
- 4 large bananas, cut into slices width ways
- 1/3 cup packed brown sugar
- 30g butter
- 1 cup heavy cream
- 1 scoop vanilla ice cream per serving

**Method:**
1. Press the MEAT/CHICKEN button on your PPC-XL.
2. Add the butter to the pot and heat until melted.
3. Add the brown sugar and heat until just dissolved.
4. Whisk the cream into the butter and sugar, keep whisking while the mixture heats, until thick.
5. Add the banana slices to the pot and stir into the caramel, let the mixture simmer for a minute or until the bananas are soft and hot.
6. Spoon the bananas and sauce over the ice cream and serve immediately.
7. ENJOY!

## *Vanilla custard*

*Custard can be enjoyed on its own for a simple dessert, or served as a side with cake, fruit, or steamed pudding.*

**Serves:** makes 1 large jug of custard, about 6 servings
**Time:** approximately 20 minutes

**Ingredients:**
- 1 ¼ cups cream
- ¾ cup full fat milk
- 4 egg yolks
- 3tsp vanilla extract
- 1/3 cup sugar

**Method:**
1. In a medium bowl, whisk the egg yolks, sugar, and vanilla together until smooth and pale.
2. While whisking, pour the cream and milk into the bowl and whisk until combined and smooth.
3. Press the RICE/RISOTTO button on your PPC-XL and keep the time to the default 6 minutes, (white rice setting).
4. Pour 3 cups of water into the bottom of the pot and place the bowl of custard into the water, making sure the water does not come more than half way up the bowl.
5. Secure the lid onto the pot and make sure the steam valve is closed.
6. Once the pot beeps, carefully release the steam and remove the lid.
7. Remove the bowl from the pot and stir the custard; it should be thick, smooth, and velvety.
8. ENJOY!

## *Stewed stone fruits with cinnamon and vanilla*

*Use any stone fruits you have. Peaches, nectarines, and plums are ideal for this recipe. Use a mixture of fruits if you can! This is a great accompaniment with ice cream or yoghurt for dessert, or on oatmeal for breakfast.*

**Serves:** makes 1 large bowl of stewed fruits, about 8 servings
**Time:** approximately 70 minutes

### Ingredients:
- 4 ½ lb stone fruit, skin on, cut into fifths
- 2 tsp ground cinnamon
- 3 tsp vanilla extract
- ½ cup sugar
- 1 lemon

### Method:
1. Press the SOUP/STEW button on your PPC-XL and adjust the time to 60 minutes.
2. Place the fruit, sugar, vanilla, cinnamon, juice of 1 lemon, and 1 ½ liters of water into the pot and stir.
3. Secure the lid onto the pot and make sure the steam valve is closed.
4. Once the pot beeps, carefully release the steam and remove the lid.
5. Stir the stewed fruits, place into a bowl, leave to cool, and store in the fridge with a lid or plastic wrap.
6. ENJOY!

## *Rice pudding*

*Rice pudding is a very old-fashioned dessert, but its appeal has endured because it is so deliciously creamy! The Power Pressure Cooker XL makes rice pudding an easy and fuss-free dessert to whip up any time.*

**Serves:** 6
**Time:** approximately 25 minutes

**Ingredients:**
- 1 ½ cups white rice, (Arborio, ideally)
- 1 cup full fat milk
- 1 cup cream
- ½ cup sugar
- 2 tsp vanilla extract

**Method:**
1. Press the RICE/RISOTTO button on your PPC-XL and keep the time at the default 6 minutes (white rice setting).
2. Pour the rice and 2 cups of water into the pot and stir.
3. Secure the lid onto the pot and make sure the steam valve is closed.
4. Once the pot beeps, carefully release the steam and remove the lid, stir the rice.
5. Press the MEAT/CHICKEN button on your PPC-XL.
6. Add the cream, milk, sugar, and vanilla to the pot and stir to combine with the rice.
7. Stir the rice mixture as it thickens to your liking.
8. Serve hot, warm, or cold.
9. ENJOY!

## Simple cheesecake

*This is a no-brainer! Cheesecake is one of the world's best culinary creations, and you'll be pleased to know it can be made in the Power Pressure Cooker XL! This is a very simple cheesecake recipe, but you can brighten it with berries when serving!*

**Serves:** 8 - 10
**Time:** approximately 40 minutes

**Ingredients:**
- 250g plain biscuits, (vanilla flavored biscuits are fine), crushed
- 150g butter, melted
- 500g cream cheese, room temperature
- 2 eggs
- ½ cup sugar

**Method:**
1. Mix together the crushed biscuits and melted butter until a wet, sandy texture forms.
2. Press the biscuit mixture into a greased, round tin, (preferably spring form).
3. With an electric beater, beat together the cream cheese, eggs, and sugar in a large bowl until combined and smooth.
4. Pour the cream cheese mixture on top of the biscuit base.
5. Press the RICE/RISOTTO button on your PPC-XL and adjust the time to 25 minutes, (wild rice setting).
6. Pour 2 cups of water into the bottom of the pot and place a trivet into the pot.
7. Carefully lower the cheesecake tin into the pot and sit it on top of the trivet.
8. Secure the lid and make sure the steam valve is closed.
9. Once the pot beeps, carefully release the steam and remove the lid.
10. Take the cheesecake out of the pot and leave it on the bench to cool and set for a further hour.
11. Serve with fresh berries and cream.
12. ENJOY!

## *Citrus pie*

*I have a confession…lemony desserts are my favorite…even more so than chocolate! Don't judge me. This pie is crazily simple, yet so tangy and delicious, you'll want the whole thing to yourself.*

**Serves:** 8 – 10
**Time:** approximately 30 minutes

**Ingredients:**
- 250g plain biscuits, crushed
- 150g butter, melted
- 2 tins condensed milk, (about 700gm give or take)
- 3 ripe lemons
- 3 egg yolks

**Method:**
1. In a large bowl, mix together the crushed biscuits and melted butter until a wet, sandy texture forms.
2. Press the biscuit mixture into a greased tin (preferably spring form).
3. In a bowl, whisk together the condensed milk, rind and juice of 2 lemons, and egg yolks.
4. Pour the lemon filling mixture onto the biscuit base.
5. Press the RICE/RISOTTO button on your PPC-XL and adjust the time to 18 minutes, (brown rice setting).
6. Pour 2 cups of water into the pot and place a trivet into the pot.
7. Carefully place the pie tin in the pot, on top of the trivet.
8. Secure the lid onto the pot and make sure the steam valve is closed.
9. Once the pot beeps, allow the steam to release on its own, and then remove the lid.
10. Sit the pie on the bench for about an hour to cool and set, before removing from the tin to slice and serve.
11. ENJOY!

## *Salted caramel sauce*

*Salted caramel is so very trendy these days, and I am ALL for it! Salty-sweet has always been a great flavor profile, as it tantalizes so many taste buds. I like to serve this sauce over vanilla ice cream.*

**Serves:** Makes 1 large jar of sauce, about 12 small servings
**Time:** approximately 12 minutes

## Ingredients:
- 2 cups cream
- 200g butter
- 1 cup sugar
- 1 tsp sea salt (or ½ teaspoon table salt)

## Method:
1. Press the MEAT/CHICKEN button on your PPC-XL.
2. Place the cream, butter, and sugar into the pot and stir gently as the butter melts and the sugar dissolves.
3. Once all ingredients have dissolved, use a whisk to keep the sauce moving as it thickens.
4. Once the sauce has reached a thick, pourable consistency, stir the salt in until dissolved.
5. Taste the sauce to see if there's enough salty flavor for your liking, and add more if need be.
6. Pour into a clean jar and keep in the fridge with the lid on.
7. Use as you wish.
8. ENJOY!

## *Ginger pudding*

*This dessert always reminds me of a friend of mine, as her Grandma makes her a ginger pudding every Christmas, just for her! I don't have that particular recipe...so I had to make it up and hope for the best! I assure you, it's delicious.*

**Serves:** 6-8
**Time:** approximately 40 minutes

**Ingredients:**
- 150g butter, softened
- ½ cup sugar
- 1 ½ cups self-raising flour
- 2 tsp ground ginger
- 2/3 cup milk

**Method:**
1. With an electric egg beater, beat the butter and sugar in a large bowl until pale and fluffy.
2. Sift the flour and ginger into the bowl and stir until just combined.
3. Add the milk to the bowl and stir until just combined, be careful not to overwork the mixture.
4. Grease a pudding basin or steamed pudding tin with butter.
5. If you want to, you can add ½ cup of golden syrup into the bottom of the tin for a decadent surprise.
6. Pour the pudding mixture into the tin and secure the lid closed. If the tin doesn't have a lid, use 2 sheets of baking paper as a lid, and secure it with string around the outer rim of the tin.
7. Press the MEAT/CHICKEN button on your PPC-XL and adjust the time to 40 minutes.
8. Place a trivet into the pot and place the pudding tin onto the trivet.
9. Pour 4 cups of hot water into the pot (don't let the water come past halfway up the tin).
10. Secure the lid onto the pot and make sure the steam valve is closed.
11. Once the pot beeps, carefully release the steam and remove the lid.
12. Remove the tin from the pot and serve the pudding while hot, with cream, custard, or ice cream.
13. ENJOY!

## *Pear crumble*

*Crumble just has to be one of the best desserts ever. If you don't have pears, or they are not currently in season, use any fruit you like! Apple and berries, peaches and plums...these are just some of the great combinations you could try.*

**Serves:** 6-8
**Time:** approximately 20 minutes

**Ingredients:**
- 6 large pears, peeled, cored, and sliced
- 200g butter, cold, cubed
- 2 cups plain flour
- 1 cup brown sugar
- 1 tsp cinnamon

**Method:**
1. In a large bowl, mix together the flour, cinnamon, and sugar.
2. Add the butter cubes to the bowl and rub the butter into the dry ingredients with your fingers until the mixture resembles crumbs and there are no large chunks of butter left.
3. Take a round dish (make sure it fits in the PPC-XL), and place the sliced pears inside. Sprinkle with 2tbsp water, and some extra cinnamon and brown sugar.
4. Sprinkle the crumble over the pears.
5. Press the SOUP/STEW button on the PPC-XL and keep the time at the default 10 minutes, place a trivet into the pot.
6. Pour 2 cups of water into the pot.
7. Place the crumble dish onto the trivet, secure the lid onto the pot, and make sure the steam valve is closed.
8. Once the pot beeps, carefully release the steam and remove the lid.
9. Serve with vanilla ice cream.
10. ENJOY!

## *Baked apples*

*When apples are "baked" with brown sugar, butter, and raisins, they turn into a rich, sweet, and caramelized treat. Serve with vanilla ice cream or plain, thick yoghurt for a wholesome dessert.*

**Serves:** makes 6 apples, (1 apple per serving)
**Time:** approximately 15 minutes

### Ingredients:
- 6 apples, (any apples you have, I use Granny Smith if they're available)
- ½ cup brown sugar
- 2 tsp cinnamon
- 50g butter, cut into 6 pieces
- ½ cup raisins

### Method:
1. Core the apples with an apple corer.
2. In a small bowl, combine the sugar, cinnamon, and raisins.
3. Place the cored apples in the PPC-XL and fill each apple with the brown sugar mixture, and place a knob of butter on top of each apple, sprinkle the remaining sugar mixture over the top of the apples.
4. Pour 1 cup of water into the pot, around the base of the apples (not over the top, as it will dissolve the sugar).
5. Press the SOUP/STEW button on the PPC-XL and keep the time to the default 10 minutes.
6. Secure the lid onto the pot and make sure the steam valve is closed.
7. Once the pot beeps, carefully release the steam and remove the lid.
8. Serve the apples with a drizzle of sauce poured over the top.
9. ENJOY!

## *Lemon curd (for drizzling and topping)*

Lemon curd is such a handy and versatile treat to have in the fridge. You can pour it over yoghurt or ice cream, or use it as a tangy filling for cakes. If you have excess lemons on the tree, try this recipe!

**Serves:** 2 medium jars of curd
**Time:** approximately 20 minutes

**Ingredients:**
- 90g butter, softened
- 1 cup sugar
- 2 eggs
- 2 egg yolks
- ¾ cup fresh lemon juice
- Zest of 2 whole lemons

**Method:**
1. In a bowl, whisk the butter and sugar vigorously until the sugar has almost dissolved and the mixture is smooth.
2. Add the eggs, yolks, lemon zest, and lemon juice, whisk until combined.
3. Pour the mixture into 2 medium jars and secure the lids on.
4. Press the BEANS/LENTILS button on the PPC-XL and adjust the time to 15 minutes.
5. Pour 2 cups of water into the pot, and place a trivet into the bottom of the pot.
6. Place the jars on the trivet, secure the lid closed, and make sure the steam valve is closed.
7. Once the pot beeps, carefully release the steam and remove the lid.
8. Leave the jars in the pot for about 20 minutes to cool.
9. Remove the jars, take the lids off, stir the curd, and store in the fridge.
10. ENJOY!

## *Mini berry cheesecakes*

*I just had to include another cheesecake recipe, as they're so delicious. These mini cheesecakes include beautiful berries to freshen the palate. This cheesecake doesn't have a base, so it's great for those who follow a gluten-free diet.*

**Serves:** makes 6 mini cheesecakes
**Time:** approximately 30 minutes

### Ingredients:
- 500g cream cheese, room temperature
- 2 eggs
- 2tsp vanilla extract
- ½ cup sugar
- 1 cup fresh berries, (use any berries you like)

### Method:
1. In a large bowl, beat together the cream cheese, eggs, vanilla, and sugar with an egg beater until smooth.
2. Fold the fresh berries into the cheesecake mixture.
3. Grease 6 ramekins with butter, and pour the cheesecake mixture into each ramekin.
4. Press the RICE/RISOTTO button on your PPC-XL and adjust the time to 25 minutes, (wild rice setting).
5. Pour 2 cups of water into the bottom of the pot and place a trivet into the pot.
6. Carefully place the ramekins onto the trivet.
7. Secure the lid and make sure the steam valve is closed.
8. Once the pot beeps, carefully release the steam and remove the lid.
9. Take the cheesecakes out of the pot and leave them on the bench to cool and set for a further hour.
10. ENJOY!

# Conclusion

Here we are, at the end of this epic recipe journey! I hope you have enjoyed these recipes, and have found a few new favorites to create every week.

Eating healthy and delicious meals does not have to be expensive, time consuming, and complicated. These recipes prove this point, as they have no more than 5 ingredients…and they're all super easy to throw together! I believe in simple, easy food, and the Power Pressure Cooker XL is a huge help in achieving this.

Thank you for coming on this delicious journey with me. I hope you have fun experimenting with your PPC-XL, and that you use my recipes as a jumping-off point!

## Resources:

While all of these recipes are my own variations and creations, I turned to the Power Pressure Cooker XL website for help and guidance when needed!

Thank you to the Power Pressure Cooker XL website for their comprehensive information and pressure cooking tips.

http://www.powerpressurecooker.com/

Pressure Cooking Today is a great resource for when you get stuck and need a few tips and tricks to keep up your sleeve.

https://www.pressurecookingtoday.com/

Printed by Libri Plureos GmbH in Hamburg, Germany